A CRY
EVER

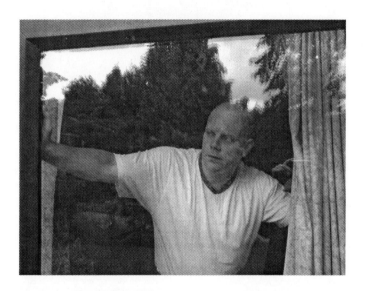

BY STEPHEN DRAKE

'One million people commit suicide every year'
The World Health Organization

Published by
Chipmunkapublishing
PO Box 6872
Brentwood
Essex CM13 1ZT
United Kingdom

http://www.chipmunkapublishing.com

A CRY FOR EVER

Chapter 1

Charlie had a settled routine. Most evenings he sat with Linda in her cramped flat. They were two people thrown together, more by circumstances than choice.

"If I didn't have these intrusive thoughts," he pondered, glancing at his dumpy companion, "I'd much rather be down the pub."

Meanwhile, Linda was thinking, "Wish I could get out more. Most girls my age don't have to sit in, night after night, looking after two kids."

Daytime was just as exciting: Charlie had therapy walks with Colin.

"If only I was normal," mused Charlie, walking along the road, hands swinging freely. "It's bad enough with Colin, but I can't imagine how bad it would be without him. I'm trying to beat the unwanted ideas by walking in public - at least it gives me a reason to get out. But as for Colin........ what a friend!"

Each week, usually on a Tuesday, Charlie attended his appointment with Dr. King.

"Not been too bad, this week," he said to the psychiatrist, "the sulpiride really helps. Without those tablets, well…. I just ain't sure."

Wednesday, mid-morning, Colin and Charlie headed for the local shops. Therapy walks: a necessary evil.

"Is anyone there?" Charlie asked his mate, trying to keep calm.

"Nobody near. Everything's fine."

They walked and talked.

Minutes later, horror of horrors, an elderly couple hobbled into view.

"Come on," urged Charlie, "you can do it."

He glanced at Colin; he didn't want to face this alone.

"I'd rather walk past twenty skinheads," he pondered, "than face this couple."

He made it past….. at a cost.

"Did I do anything strange?" he asked, desperately trying not to panic.

"Nothing at all," replied Colin, "and I didn't take my eyes off you for a second."

The therapy walk was not a success.

"That's the worst the intrusions have been since I've been taking my new tablets," thought Charlie, as he plodded into his mother's house, closely followed by Colin.

"Fancy going out tonight?" asked Colin, unaware of his friend's anxiety.

He lifted the kettle and held it under the tap.

"I know a nice little bar. Wall-to-wall totty."

"I ain't sure," replied Charlie, "my nerves are so bad at the moment. I feel really shagged off!"

"Then a good night on the town is just what you need. And don't worry, I won't leave your side."

"Okay, then."

The wine bar heaved to the beat of unfamiliar tunes. Smartly-dressed,

well-spoken clientele mingled.

"All trying to impress," thought Charlie, feeling uneasy in his denim dungarees.

"I really find it difficult to relax in public, especially in places like this," he thought, watching a suited gent try his luck with a skinny waitress.

"Don't think he'll get lucky," Charlie decided, gauging her reaction.

"What do you reckon?" Colin yelled, struggling to be heard above the steady beat.

"It's good," shouted Charlie, trying to convey enthusiasm he didn't really feel.

"I must try and make the most of it," thought Charlie, "just so Colin can have a good time."

"Look at the talent," screamed Colin, "seen anything you like?"

"Plenty," responded Charlie, "but I am with somebody."

"So; it's never worried you before."

Charlie glanced around the bar.

"Lots of posh, older women," he mused, "maybe......"

Charlie had paid little, if any, attention to the male clientele.

"You got a problem?"

Charlie was taken completely by surprise. He looked at the man standing in front of him. Smart but casual, aged in his thirties, slightly built, average height and steaming drunk.

"Must have a point to prove," he decided, "why couldn't he have proved it to someone else? I really don't need this. I'm only here for Colin."

"Do you want a problem?" Charlie responded, reluctant to take things further.

It took all the drunkard's effort to remain upright.

"He hasn't got a clue what he's doing," thought Charlie, "trust my luck! If it ain't intrusive thoughts then it's some tosser having a dig."

Colin jumped between the two men.

"Leave it, Charlie," he ordered, "it ain't worth the effort. This bloke can hardly walk."

"Okay mate," said Charlie.

Charlie glanced at Colin. The drunkard swayed, looking bemused.

"This is shit," thought Charlie, "can rarely get out and when I do....."

Colin stepped aside.

"Why not?" Charlie thought, angry with his intrusions, life in general, quite a few things, but not particularly the drunkard.

Charlie's bald head crashed into the drunkard's nose. The blood dripped steadily to the floor. The man was bent double, desperately trying not to collapse.

"Oh shit," said Charlie, panicking, realising he had an audience.

"You bloody idiot," bawled Colin, "what the hell did you do that for?"

It wasn't long before the bouncers made an unwelcome appearance. A cropped-haired, burly, tattooed thug in a dinner suit lunged at Charlie. Colin, bravely, stood between his pal and the bouncer.

"Don't worry, mate," yelled Colin, "I'm taking him home. Now."

"You better fucking had!"

Colin led Charlie from the wine bar. They clambered into Colin's car and hit the road.

"There wasn't any need for that, was there?" Colin groaned.

"No, mate. I'm sorry." Charlie replied.

"I need to get my head together," he thought, "or things will only get worse."

Days later, on a boring Thursday evening, Charlie and Linda were watching a documentary about some poor sod with depression who kept trying to harm himself.

"Poor bastard," thought Charlie, "trouble is, it's so bloody common."

Footsteps could be heard outside. Then, there was a short, sharp tap on the window.

"Who the hell is that?" Linda snapped, "look at the fucking time."

Charlie jumped to his feet, glad of the interruption. He pulled the dirty grey curtains.

"Hello Colbo" he said, opening the window, "is everything okay?"

"Can we talk?" said Colin, looking at Linda, "In private."

"Yeah, course," answered Charlie.

"Just going out for a while," he said, turning to Linda.

She scowled.

Charlie jumped out of the window and joined his pal. They ambled along the empty street; nothing was said.

"Let's sit here," said Colin, breaking the silence, indicating a brick wall.

"What's happened?" asked Charlie.

"Well" began Colin, "do you remember me talking about Guy Henderson? I've known him for years. Thought we were really good mates. Anyway, he asked me for some money as he'd heard about a car for sale. He said it was a brilliant deal and he shouldn't hang about. I gave him the money and I ain't seen him since."

"What a bastard," said Charlie, "how much did you give him?"

"Eight grand."

"Any idea where he's gone?" asked Charlie.

"No. I'll try to find him, but I ain't got a clue."

"If I can do anything, let me know."

The two men sat and talked.

"Colin is really low," thought Charlie, "I've never seen him like this."

"Look," he said, "why don't you stay at my place tonight? Hazel won't mind."

"Okay, thanks."

They retraced their steps to Linda's flat. She hadn't bothered to shut the window.

"Me and Colin are going back to my place," yelled Charlie.

"That's great," said Linda, "thanks for another lovely evening."

"Sarcastic trollop," thought Charlie, heading for home.

Charlie lay on his bed, while Colin settled for an old, lumpy mattress on the floor.

They talked, about nothing in particular.

"Out of ten, how would you rate Linda for personality and looks?" Colin asked.

"He seems much brighter," thought Charlie, "hope he can just forget about his money."

He cleared his throat.

"Personality - flawless. Looks - full marks."

"If you weren't dating her?" continued Colin.

"Personality - grumpy, moody, hasn't really got one. Looks - decidedly lacking. Wish I could do better."

Colin laughed.

The chatter began to fade. A competition for staying awake longest followed.

"So, who's the best bird you've been with? I don't mean looks and personality..... the best performer," whispered Charlie.

There was no answer, except soft, regular breathing .

"Have a good sleep, mate" murmured Charlie, "nobody needs this shit, but it'll be okay."

Charlie pulled the duvet over his head and tried to sleep. His body was tired but his mind was fully alert.

"Oh, to be loaded," he mused, "then I could give Colin his money back. Still, I don't think it's only the money; it's also that his mate has conned him. Taken him for a right prick."

He fell asleep.... eventually.

He rolled over and peered at the clock through squinted eyes.

"Six-thirty," he mumbled, "for fuck's sake."

He closed his eyes; it certainly wasn't healthy to start the day at such an unearthly hour.

The night before came flooding back...... Colin.

The mattress lay on the floor - empty. The window had been opened and the orange curtains moved gently with the

breeze.
"Shit."

Charlie was fully awake. Adrenalin is stronger than any coffee.
"What the hell should I do?" Charlie murmured.
Feelings of anxiety gripped him.
"I'll phone him at home," decided Charlie, "in a bit."
His heart raced and his breathing was rapid and shallow.
"No need to panic," he thought, trying to regain some sort of composure, "he's probably gone for a walk to clear his head."

Charlie walked into the kitchen and filled the kettle. He rang Colin's number.
 "Come on," he muttered, "just answer the bloody phone."
Charlie kept trying, religiously, throughout the day. Finally, his patience was rewarded.
"Hello."
Colin lived at home with his mother, brother and step-father, Paul. The gruff tone was familiar.
"Hello, Paul," said Charlie, "can I have a word with Colin?"
"I'll go and look in his room. I'm not sure if he's here."
Charlie waited. What could have only been a few seconds seemed like hours.
"Hello Charlie," said Paul, "he's not about. When I see him I'll tell him you called."
"Okay, thanks."

That day was an emotional rollercoaster.
"I've nothing to worry about," pondered Charlie, "Colin was quite happy when he left. There ain't a problem."
The lows, inevitably, followed.
"You weren't much of a friend. He obviously had a lot on his mind and you didn't really help."
It had been dark for hours. Charlie, with no other options, headed for bed.
He tossed and turned. He lay under the cover, then on top. He stared into the darkness, then he closed his eyes and tried to empty his mind. Nothing worked. Finally, he heard the birds outside his window, happily singing at the start of a new day.

A CRY FOR EVER

There was a soft, almost apologetic, knock on the back door. Charlie struggled into a sitting position, rubbing his eyes. He couldn't have been asleep for more than an hour.

His mother opened the door. He heard voices.

"It must be Colin," thought Charlie, "fucking pucker!"

Footsteps could be heard along the hallway before the bedroom door swung open.

No Colin!

Paul and Alan, Colin's step-dad and brother; Edward and Julian, friends of Charlie; and Linda trudged into the room. They stood around Charlie's bed. Nothing was said for what seemed like an eternity.

Edward, staring at the floor, finally spoke.

"We've got some ….. um…….. very bad news," he stammered.

"Oh," said Charlie, "surely it ain't that bad."

"It's Colin," continued Edward, "he's killed himself."

Time froze. The words hung in the air.

Charlie's thoughts were confused.

"Not sunk in….. hasn't registered……can't comprehend…… must be a mistake….."

He looked at each person. Nobody uttered a word. He had been six when he first experienced death – of his beloved cat, Penny. It felt like his world had ended. But this was worse, much worse. He felt like a child now, with no control in an adult world. He acted on his feelings, covering his shaven head with his duvet. He wanted to stay like this forever. But he had to live, starting now. He peered from under the duvet, eyes flickering but dry. No tears…. yet.

"What exactly happened?" he asked, voice quivering.

"He gassed himself in his car. His body was found early this morning," said Edward, outwardly calm.

Charlie flinched.

"We found this letter in his room," said Paul, in a level tone, "some of it is for you."

Paul handed Charlie a piece of paper, covered with untidy scrawl.

Charlie stared at the note. It took a while for him to focus on his mate's writing.

"Colin wrote this knowing what he intended to do," he thought, "I just can't imagine writing to people knowing that a couple of hours later.......'

The beginning of Colin's note addressed his mum and brother. He confirmed his love for them, assured them he knew exactly what he was doing and this was what he wanted. He asked their forgiveness. Charlie continued reading. The last part of the note was written for him.

"You're the best friend I could have had....."

Charlie opted not to finish. Losing control would be very undignified. Also, a solitary tear in each eye was blurring his vision.

He handed back the note. He hoped nobody would notice the slight tremor in his hand.

"Can I have a copy?" he asked.

No-one wanted to say the wrong thing, but nearly everyone felt they should say something. Not Charlie and Alan. Conversation was just a step too far. Alan sat, back against the wall, with his head in his hands and tears in his eyes. Charlie, still on the bed, stared at the ceiling.

"I can't believe it" thought Charlie, "I just can't fucking believe it. Why Colin? Of all the fuckers in this world - why him?"

Linda decided it would be best not to leave Charlie alone. She was like a shadow. Charlie sat at the kitchen table, staring into the garden. He didn't see the trees or flowers, or hear the birds. His mind was elsewhere..... in the past, when Colin had filled his life. Linda made a phone call.

"I've got a babysitter for tonight, so I'll be able to stay," she said.

"Okay," replied Charlie, not bothered in the least, but reluctant to argue.

It was approaching midnight when Charlie and Linda opted for bed. Charlie lay, eyes wide open, staring into the darkness. Sleep wasn't really an option.

"I just can't sleep," he said, "so I'm going for a walk."

"I'll come with you," offered Linda.

"No. I'd rather be alone."

Charlie plodded aimlessly, hour after hour. Time meant nothing. In fact, nothing on Earth meant anything to him as he trudged the deserted roads. He passed the clubhouse belonging to Effingham golf course.

"Spent an evening in there with Colin," recalled Charlie. "He was in good form that night. Only two women in the club. Must have been about fifty men. Still, he wasn't gonna let that stop him. He certainly wasn't put off easily. I'm sure they were lying about having a social disease."

He must have walked miles in the freezing cold. His hands were numb but he really didn't care.

"What about that black girl Colin dated," recalled Charlie, "she was gorgeous, but he left her for a fat little tart with a spotty arse just 'cause she liked his tattoo."

A car passed; the first sign of life since Charlie had started walking.

"Colin really was a great mate," he thought, "who else would spend every spare minute helping me with therapy? Nothing was too much trouble. He was too nice for this poxy world, anyway."

A tear trickled down his cheek.

"I can't imagine his pain as he wrote that suicide note," agonised Charlie.

The floodgates opened. He sat at the side of the road and sobbed. He ached; it was a physical pain. Life could never be the same.It took a long time and much effort for Charlie to regain some sort of composure.

Dawn was beginning to break. Charlie, with heavy heart and swollen eyes, trudged homewards. The birds sang from the trees. The dew formed on the grass. Everything was, in fact, as normal.

"Colin.....why?" questioned Charlie, picturing his friend's smiling face.

"Colin's car; hosepipe; fumes; suffering; death," wiped away any smiles.

Charlie shook as he fought to dispel the repulsive images.

As quietly as possible, he opened the back door. As he expected, all the occupants were fast asleep. He crept into the bedroom, taking great care not to disturb Linda.

"I certainly don't need her giving me the third degree," he decided.

He found a blanket in the wardrobe and a cushion on the chair. He lay on the floor and prayed for some sleep. Eventually, after many disturbing images, his prayers were answered.

Chapter 2

When Charlie stirred, it was almost midday.
"Why the hell am I on the floor?" he moaned.
It only took a split second for reality to strike.
"Colin...... oh fuck," he muttered.
He clambered to his feet.
"I've got to get up sometime, so it might as well be now."
A piece of crumpled paper, covered in scruffy writing, rested on the chair.
"Didn't want to wake you. Ring me if you need anything. See you tonight. Linda"
He tossed the note onto the floor and headed for the kitchen.

"It's gonna be bloody awful without Colin," he pondered, "the days are just gonna drag on and on."
He slumped at the kitchen table.
"Longer days, fewer visits, niggling thoughts, feeling depressed. Hope I don't get any intrusive ideas."
Charlie made a coffee and rolled a cigarette.
"What if I do get the bastard intrusions," he pondered, "I don't deserve to be happy. Colin, one of the nicest people you could meet, was so fucked off that he killed himself. If <u>he</u> didn't deserve to be happy....... then, who does? Certainly not me."

The phone shrilled, providing a welcome distraction.
"Hello mate, it's Ed."
"What's happening?" asked Charlie.
"Not much. Feeling totally gutted."
"Same here," said Charlie, trying to hide any emotions, "I just can't believe it. It hasn't sunk in. Don't think it ever will."
They chatted for a while.
"I'd better go," said Edward, "I'll try and pop round later. If I can't, I'll call you."
"Okay, mate," said Charlie, "take care."
He kept hold of the phone, as if trying to find comfort from the dialling tone, but it didn't work.

Charlie hadn't left the house for nearly two days. Even a stroll in the garden seemed daunting.
"I must make an effort to get out and about," he urged

12

himself, "or I'll be stuck in this house forever."

He was only too aware that the longer he stayed inside, the harder it would be.

"That's it," he decided, "I'm going to walk to the shop. It ain't far, so it should be easy. I'm still taking my tablets, so I reckon I'll be okay."

As he took his denim jacket from the hook, he felt a familiar unease. Heart rate slightly too rapid and stomach slightly knotted.

He left the house and headed towards the nearest shop. He trudged along, trying to stay calm and focused.

"Was there an old woman? Have I hurt her?"

Charlie was completely shocked by the sudden intrusion.

"Shit. What the fuck!"

He, quickly and intently, studied his surroundings. There was no-one to be seen. He tried not to panic, but the situation was beyond his control. He clasped his hands and stood still, frozen to the spot. His heart pounded and his breathing was shallow and rapid.

"Mustn't completely lose it," he thought.

His head spun like a drunkard after a heavy night.

"Oh no," he moaned, "where the fuck did that come from? Hell. How will I cope without Colin?"

Utter despair! He dreaded, even feared, the future.

It was at least fifteen minutes before he had the confidence to move.

"Fuck the shop," he decided, "I'm going home."

Charlie stomped into the house, went straight to his bedroom and flung himself onto the unmade bed.

"Bad….. bad….bad," he cursed, "I don't believe this is happening."

He hadn't been lying on the bed for very long when the shrill of the phone disturbed him. His bald head left the pillow.

"Bollocks," he thought, "I really can't face anyone now."

The phone rang a few times during the next couple of hours.

"Somebody is desperate to talk," thought Charlie, "and, unfortunately, I can't lie here, forever."

Finally, he answered the phone.

"Hello," he said.

"Hello, it's Paul. I wanted to let you know that Colin's funeral will be held in Fetcham, this Friday at eleven o'clock. Please tell anyone you feel ought to be there."

"Thanks," said Charlie, "I will."

He went straight back to his room and lay on the bed.

"The church is going to be packed," he thought, feeling a sense of unease, "I just know the intrusions will cause me so much hassle."

Rolling a cigarette proved tricky in the horizontal position.

"Whatever happens," he decided, "I'll be there."

The sun shone, but a sharp chill filled the air.

"Colin's funeral," pondered Charlie, staring out the window, "at least it ain't raining. I still can't believe he's actually gone."

"It's time to go," called Charlie's mother, "are you ready?"

"Yeah," he replied, coming out the bathroom.

"You're not wearing dungarees, are you?" Hazel asked, looking at her son.

"Course I am," replied Charlie, "I certainly don't think Colin would have had a problem about it."

Linda and Edward were already at the church when Charlie and his mother arrived.

"Feel gutted," said Edward, "he was so young. Never knew he was so depressed."

"Terrible," answered Charlie, "don't think I'll ever get over it."

Many family and friends stood outside the church. Hushed chatter, nervous laughter and stifled sobs. Complete silence fell as Colin completed his final journey.

The crying and hugging continued long after the service had finished.

Every week, Charlie kept his appointment with Dr. King. These appointments, together with his medication, provided a lifeline.

"How much sulpiride are you taking?" Dr. King asked.

"Twelve tablets," answered Charlie.

"200mg each?"

"I think so," answered Charlie.

"Well," said the doctor, "that is much too high a dose. We must reduce the amount and, eventually, stop it completely."

"Why's that?" asked Charlie, "I'd rather keep taking it. I know that it helps."

"Being on sulpiride for too long can be physically damaging

14

to you. There are many unpleasant conditions associated with long-term use of the drug."

"Oh," said Charlie.

"So, we'll start by reducing your dose to ten tablets daily. Okay?"

"Too bad if it's not okay," thought Charlie, leaving the surgery.

He joined his mother in the waiting room.

"I really hope that I can manage without my tablets," he pondered, following his mother to the car.

Charlie sat at the kitchen table, coffee in one hand and roll-up in the other.

"Colin has been dead for over a month and I still can't move on," he thought, "intrusions are bad so I rarely go out alone in the daytime, feel shit...... oh fuck, what's the point?"

It was a frosty evening, mimicking Linda's mood. Charlie sat in her flat, watching a comedy on BBC2. He had stopped trying to make conversation with Linda, it'd be easier finding a cure for OCD."

"Going to bed," said Linda, "what you doing?"

"I'll go home," said Charlie, struggling to his feet.

He headed towards the door.

"Should be okay," thought Charlie, "it'll take me about forty minutes to get home but, at this time of night, I won't bump into any old women. I'm sure it'll be fine."

Charlie stared at Dr. King. The doctor returned his gaze.

"It's been a few months since we began to reduce your medication," said Dr. King, "I really believe it's the right time to try and manage without any sulpiride. Would you be happy to try?"

"I suppose so," answered Charlie, "if you really think I'll be ok."

After two days in the pill-free zone, Charlie was pleased to report no major upsets. He sat at the kitchen table staring into the garden.

"It's not raining," he thought, "reckon I should try and get out during the day. Even without my pills, I'm sure I'll be ok."

As he plodded along the road, he tried to think positively.

"There's no-one about, I'll be fine."

A figure turned into the lane. Charlie walked forward, slightly uneasy but determined not to be beaten. It wasn't long before he had a good view of the other person.

"Oh no," he panicked, "I don't believe it."

The old lady, walking stick in one hand and pulling a shopping bag with the other, struggled towards the young man. She couldn't possibly have imagined the stress her presence caused.

"Calm down," he urged, "she's one hundred metres away, at least."

Charlie stopped walking. His heart-rate and breathing rate had increased. His mouth felt dry and he noticed a throbbing pain on one side of his head.

"Look," he murmured, "you've done well. You've been out, during the day, without any pills. Go home now and try again another day. There's no point trying to walk past that lady and making yourself ill."

As he turned towards home, away from the old lady, his anxiety levels dropped dramatically.

"She's miles away," he reassured himself, "you certainly ain't harmed her."

He raced back to the house, desperate for its security.

Charlie flicked channels but could find nothing of interest. He glanced at Linda. She looked as bored as he felt.

"I think I'll go to bed," she yawned, "I'm knackered. What you doing?"

"I'll make a move," said Charlie, "call me tomorrow."

He quietly closed the front door, taking great care not to disturb the sleeping children.

"This'll be easy," he thought, "no problem."

He strolled, with a new-found confidence, along the dark, empty roads.

"Maybe the worst is behind me," he pondered, "could I have turned a corner? Maybe the intrusions won't bother me any more."

He passed a newsagents'. There was a dim light inside the shop, hopefully to deter thieves.

He walked through the car-park and passed the church hall.

"Oh shit. Was anybody there? Was there an old woman?"

The intrusion gave no warning, leaving him no chance to resist. He stood still, rooted to the spot. Several times he looked behind, to each side and to his front.

His heart pounded. The familiar symptoms, just as bad as he

remembered.

As he checked his surroundings, the anxiety eased...... slightly!

"Oh hell," he moaned, "why me? Now, I've just got to get home."

He walked on, unsteady and dejected.

He passed the playing fields, still fighting to stay in control. As he walked, without warning, his right shoulder began to droop. Gradually at first, but however hard he tried, he just couldn't straighten his upper body.

"What the fuck's happening to me," he panicked, "I've no control over my shoulder."

With his shoulder slanting unnaturally towards the pavement, Charlie struggled to move forward.

He felt a strange sensation in his right leg. Quickly, the leg became heavy and weak, making walking very difficult.

"This is serious," thought Charlie, "what next?"

His right shoulder dropped further. His leg offered no support.

"I can't feel my leg at all," he panicked, "there's no fucking sensation. It's just a dead weight."

He tried to stay upright.

"There's no way I'm going to get home like this," he thought, "I can barely move."

He looked around; nobody for miles.

"Calm down," he urged, "I'll just sit here for a while. You never know, I might be okay in a bit."

Charlie slumped to the kerb. He sat, staring into the darkness, as the minutes ticked away.

"I've given it ten minutes, at least," he decided, "I've got to try and get home."

His efforts to stand failed miserably. His right leg had no sensation and his shoulder wouldn't straighten.

"I ain't got a choice," he decided, "I'm gonna have to crawl."

A couple of miles, on hands and knees, is a long way.

"I understand why a baby screams when its rattle is at the other end of a room," thought Charlie.

It wasn't long, a matter of yards, before his knees throbbed, each movement more painful than the one before. He surveyed the damage. His dungarees were torn and blood oozed from his exposed skin. His hands were freezing, red and scratched.

"Got to have a rest," decided Charlie, anxiously looking at his knees, "I just can't go on."

He stopped, desperately resisting an urge to lie on the pavement.

"Mustn't lie down," he thought, "if I do, I'll never get up and I'll be stuck here."

A car raced along the road, music blaring.

"Here we go," thought Charlie, "at last, a car. I'm saved."

The driver must have seen Charlie, on the pavement, but didn't stop.

"Shit," Charlie cursed, "probably thought I was a drunk trying to find more booze."

The car's engine faded into the distance.

"Got to carry on," moaned Charlie, "if I don't move, I ain't gonna get back."

He crawled and crawled. His hands and knees had numbed, providing slight relief.

"I suppose it's like having a tattoo," he pondered, "at first it's bloody agony but, after a while, you can't feel so much pain."

He had been crawling for almost three hours.

"Come on," he urged, "I'm nearly there."

He flopped onto the driveway. Knees and hands scratched, bleeding, covered in dirt and gravel and a niggling pain in his lower back.

"Thank God," he murmured.

Sensation returned to his leg and his shoulder straightened. He stood with complete ease.

"Bloody hell," he cursed, "just what's happening?"

He sprinted to the back door. Such was his haste, he almost fell through the glass panels.

"Mum," he screeched, "come here, now!"

Hazel hurried from the lounge.

"What's happened?" Hazel yelled, staring at Charlie's hands and knees.

"I was walking home from Linda's," Charlie explained, "when suddenly I just couldn't walk………."

Hazel listened intently, without interrupting or passing judgement.

"You'd better get cleaned up," she said, after her son's explanation.

18

A CRY FOR EVER

Charlie soaked in a hot, soapy bath.

"Reckon I'll get some sleep," he said to his mother, "it's been one hell of a night."

Charlie went straight to his bedroom and lay on the bed.

"What's happening to me? What's going on…" he wondered. He was soon fast asleep.

The following morning, Charlie stirred, conscious of a figure on the end of his bed.

"Good morning," said Dr. King, "how are you feeling?"

The events of the previous night came flooding back.

"I've been better," answered Charlie.

"What happened?" Dr. King asked.

"I was walking home from my girlfriend's house and everything stopped working. The only way I could get home was on my hands and knees….." Charlie struggled to explain.

"I'll just check your reflexes," said Dr. King, giving Charlie a short, sharp tap just below the knee with the side of his hand.

Both knees and both elbows were checked.

"Follow my finger with your eyes," said Dr. King, moving his finger slowly across Charlie's visual field.

"Okay," he said, "now stretch out your right arm, palm facing upwards and bring the tip of your finger to your nose."

"That's fine," he said, "now sit on the chair and close your eyes. Place your right heel on your left knee and slide your heel down to your foot."

The examinations continued until the doctor was satisfied.

"Well," said Dr. King, "I can't find any physical explanation for what happened. I suggest you start taking sulpiride again, and we'll keep a very close eye on you. Ideally, I'd like to avoid sulpiride, but given the circumstances………."

"Okay then," said Charlie, "whatever you think."

Dr. King left the room. Hushed voices could be heard from the kitchen.

"I'm sure he'll be fine," said Dr. King, "now I've started the sulpiride again."

"Thank-you very much," replied Hazel.

"Any further problems," said Dr. King, "don't hesitate to give my secretary a call."

Charlie didn't really live, he just existed in a haze of antipsychotic medication.

Day after day, he sat at the kitchen table, smoking, drinking coffee and thinking.

"Colin...... wonder what he'd be doing now," he mused, "would he still feel like shit? Would he be happier?"

Charlie sipped the scalding coffee and took a long drag from his roll-up.

"I don't feel too bad," he pondered, "suppose it must be the medication."

"You've no reason to be happy," insisted a niggling voice, "not when Colin felt so bad he killed himself."

It was a cold, miserable evening........ as usual for the time of year. Charlie and Linda sat on the sofa with a scrabble board balanced between them.

"Triple word score," said Charlie, "beat that."

"I'm pregnant," she replied.

"Shit...... blimey ......"

A baby had been discussed earlier but, after no success, quickly forgotten.

"Bloody hell," thought Charlie, "I just assumed that nothing would happen after all this time."

"What do you reckon?" Linda asked.

"Wow," answered Charlie, "don't know what to say....... brilliant."

He paced the room having completely forgotten his triple word score.

"If only I could tell Colin," he pondered.

"I hope you're a better father than you were a mate."

Feelings of joy were overwhelmed by guilt.

Linda grew bigger with the passing of each day. Charlie suffered with his intrusive thoughts, but felt unable to confide in Linda.

"She's got enough to worry about," pondered Charlie, "and she doesn't understand what these intrusions do to me."

He watched as Linda swept the kitchen floor.

"Can't talk about Colin, either," he mused, "they never got on when he was alive, and she just doesn't understand how I feel."

The following eight months saw the miracle of human life.

"Where there's death, there's life," thought Charlie, gazing at Linda's swollen tummy and seeing Colin's face in his mind's eye.

Charlie and Edward stood, expectantly, outside Epsom Hospital. People bustled about, completely oblivious to the day's importance.

"Thanks so much for being here," said Charlie, "I really wouldn't be able to do this alone."

"No problem," replied Edward.

"And," thought Charlie, "I really need somebody to check the intrusions."

"Didn't you want to actually see it all happen?" asked Edward.

"No," replied Charlie, "I'm sure that Clare will be a better birth partner than me."

"They've been mates for years, ain't they?" said Edward.

Roll-up followed roll-up until Clare appeared, seemingly from nowhere.

"It's a girl," she said, beaming, "just been born."

Charlie and Edward followed Clare through the hospital 'til they reached the labour room. Linda lay, panting, on a bed. Beside the bed, in a small plastic cot, the most gorgeous creature took her first breaths.

"Congratulations, mate," murmured Edward, "magnificent."

Charlie gazed at the tiny bundle, speechless.

"Stunning," he thought, trying to empty his mind of everything except the here and now.

He failed. The harder he tried, the more he failed.

"Colin! Smiling face! Therapy walks! Best mate! Car! Hosepipe! Death!"

Charlie fidgeted nervously, desperate for reassurance.

"What the fuck's wrong with you," he asked himself, "first child, absolutely perfect, you should be dancing in the street, but no..... you can't do fuck all."

He wanted to run; run as fast and far as he could.

"She's lovely," he stammered, "really cute."

Silence!

"We'd better make a move, Ed, or we'll miss our train," muttered Charlie.

"You sure? I ain't in a rush."

"Sure. See you later, Linda."

Charlie and Edward left the hospital.

"That was bloody awful," thought Charlie, "supposed to be

the happiest time of my life, but all I want to do is go home."

Surprisingly, the train was on time.
"She's lovely," said Charlie to Lucy, his sister, and Hazel, "now I'm really tired and just want my bed."
He went straight to his room and sat, head in hands, on the bed.
"What's happened?" he mused, "where did it all go wrong? How the hell am I going to cope with any intrusions when I'm feeling so fucked off?"

Day after day, there came intrusion after intrusion.
The rain battered the kitchen window and the wind howled across the lawn. Charlie sat at the table waiting for the kettle to boil.
"The bastard intrusions have been so bad since Colin died," he thought, "I'm still taking the maximum amount of medication, so what else am I supposed to do? And, I don't think I've ever felt this shit in my whole life."
The kettle boiled. Charlie got up. He needed a drink..... and a cigarette.
"Just wish I had someone to talk to," he thought, "but if I told anyone what was going on, I'd feel such a cunt."

This particular Wednesday evening was no different from any other. Charlie and Linda sat in her flat watching television. Becky and Alan, Linda's kids, were in bed, and baby Charlotte slept peacefully.
"Got to get my life sorted," pondered Charlie.
"You're quiet again," sneered Linda, "you have got to be the most boring person on the planet."
"Sorry," mumbled Charlie, wishing she'd drop dead.
"Maybe it would be better if you lived here," she continued, "have you decided about moving in?"
"Not really," replied Charlie, "been a bit busy."
"You do fuck all," she raged, "you ain't worth a fucking wank!"
"I'll sort everything," said Charlie, not wanting to argue, "just give me time."
"Oh, piss off."
"Right" said Charlie, "I'm going home."
Charlie left the flat...... briskly.

A CRY FOR EVER

He walked the streets, very relieved nobody was about that night.

"Why should you be happy," he taunted, "you killed your friend."

"You didn't," he answered, "course you didn't."

"But you didn't do much when he needed you. He always helped you. What did you ever do for him?"

He walked past a youth club. No sign of life.

"Was there an old woman? Did you hurt her?"

Charlie stopped as if paralysed. He looked, quickly, in every direction. The area was deserted. Even so, Charlie struggled to cope.

"Oh no," he panicked, "I just don't believe this. I just wish that I had somebody with me. Everything is so pointless."

He walked behind a block of offices, hidden by a large, wooden fence. He knew they were behind the fence - he'd burgled three of them a few years earlier.

He jumped up, grabbed the top of the fence and pulled himself over.

"I really don't give a shit what happens to me," he thought.

He found a large stone quite near the fence.

"That'll do," he decided, picking up the stone.

He hurled the stone at the window. The glass shattered, breaking the night's silence.

"Shit, what a noise," thought Charlie, "still…. who cares?"

He stepped forward and pulled away the remaining fragments of glass.

"Don't want to slash myself," he pondered.

He leaned through the opening and stretched forwards.

"No need to get in the building," decided Charlie, "I can reach the fax machine and unplug it from out here."

He pulled the fax machine out the window.

"Not bad," he thought, "I reckon it's fairly new."

He walked towards the fence holding the fax machine.

"Good job the alarms didn't work," he mumbled.

He climbed the fence, just managing to keep hold of the fax machine, and
 ambled away from the offices.

"Too bloody easy," pondered Charlie, "these places ain't got a clue. Bit pointless, though: don't need a fax machine and don't reckon I'll be able to sell it."

When Charlie got home, he put the fax machine in a shed at the top of the garden and, quietly, went into the house.

"Straight to bed," he thought, "the sooner I'm asleep, the less I suffer."

Day followed day, each one seemingly longer than the one before.

One day, Charlie had just left Linda's flat; it was almost midnight. He ambled home, hands in pockets. He felt the screwdriver; he never left home without it. He walked along an alley leading to the high street. On his left, parked under a street lamp, was an old car just waiting to be robbed.

"Why not?" thought Charlie, "do something every night; this looks a good bet."

He had a quick look into the car.

"Don't think it's alarmed," he decided, "let's do it."

Charlie hesitated.

"Come on," he urged, "what the fuck have you got to lose? No old women in prison, so who cares if you get caught?"

He took the screwdriver and, quickly, forced the back window. Hardly a sound. He put his hand through the broken window and opened the door.

He climbed into the vehicle and started to search.

"Bollocks," he cursed, "nothing except the stereo. I might as well have that."

The stereo proved difficult to remove.

"Fuck it," he said, holding the damaged stereo, "this ain't worth anything. Now I've got it out, it's so fucked, it's worthless."

Charlie left the stereo on the driver's seat, climbed out of the car, shut the door and walked away.

"What a waste of time," he cursed.

He reached the end of the alley and turned left into the high street.

"Did you just hit someone...... an old woman?" Charlie panicked.

He stopped, immediately, and checked his surroundings.

"Course you didn't," he said, "what would an old lady be doing out here at this time of night?"

"Might have just wandered off," he thought, panic rising.

He didn't move. He just had to stay calm and walking would be much too demanding.

"Relax," he thought, there's nobody about. No-one at all."

A CRY FOR EVER

He looked around…. just to be sure.

"Okay," he decided, "better get going. These fucking intrusions….. I just can't cope. If only Colin was still about……"

Charlie walked along the high street, angry, frightened and upset.

"Why me….." he moaned, "what the fuck have I done to deserve this again?"

He passed an off-licence. Dim lights were glowing in the shop.

"Oh, why not," he thought, "I really couldn't care."

He smashed the window, climbed through, and headed for the counter.

"No money," he thought, "no fags….. oh shit."

The alarm screeched, a cry in the dark.

"Oh no," panicked Charlie, "what if some nutter comes down from the flat above the shop with a gun."

Charlie grabbed three bottles of whisky and went to the broken window.

"Mustn't break them," he thought, "or all this grief will be for nothing."

Charlie managed to reach the pavement, outside the shop, without spilling a drop. He trotted along the high street and, at the first opportunity, turned into a side alley, heading for home.

"That was close," he pondered, "still, I ain't gonna stop 'til I'm nicked. These bastard intrusions are making me do it, and, anyway, why should I be happy when Colin………"

Chapter 3

Charlie's evening had been, pretty much, the norm. Watched television, rowed with Linda, then left the flat. An intrusion disturbed the young man almost as soon as he left. He stood behind a shop, icy wind on his face, staring at the back door. "Here we go," he thought, "whatever happens things ain't gonna get any worse. The intrusions are completely ruining everything I do, and Colin….. well, I don't want to go the same way."

Charlie kicked the wooden door. Nothing happened. A muddy footprint but little else.

"If at first you don't succeed……" he mumbled, kicking the exact same spot.

A loud thud……… very little else.

"Bollocks," he cursed, looking for another possible entrance.

"No other way in," he decided, kicking again.

No joy!

"My foot's gonna break before this fucking door does," he moaned, "and I'm making such a noise……"

He kicked harder.

"Who gives a shit. This is nothing compared with Colin."

Everything happened so fast. Engines, tyres, breaks…..

"Oh well," thought Charlie, trotting away from the shop, "it was always gonna happen."

"Stop! Police!"

"Don't think I will," decided Charlie, "got to play the game."

The footsteps got closer…… any moment now! A hand grabbed Charlie's jacket…….. not before time.

"You're nicked, sonny," said a breathless PC, "that's you done for the night."

Charlie, back at Dorking police station, sat in an interview room opposite two suited detectives. The larger man was tall and mostly skinny, which made his huge belly look all the more obvious.

He looks pregnant," mused Charlie, "what a state."

The other detective was a short, fat and bald with an odd shaped head that resembled a boiled egg.

"Wonder if these two are married," pondered Charlie.

"I gather you won't be denying tonight's offence," began

Belly.

"No," answered Charlie, "I was trying to gain entry to the shop."

"Are there any further offences you'd like us to consider?" asked Egg-head.

"Um......" began Charlie.

"Well," said Egg-head, "the drinking club by the recreation ground, was that you?"

"Yeah," replied Charlie, "it was."

"So, what did you take?"

"I got cash from the fruit machines," said Charlie, "and cigarettes from behind the bar."

"And," continued Egg-head, "a house was burgled along Lower Road. Was that you?"

"No," answered Charlie, "I don't burgle houses."

"Right," said Belly, "there was a break-in at the golf club. Do you know anything about that?"

"Yeah," replied Charlie, "that was me, too."

Belly and Egg-head enjoyed a very successful couple of hours.

"They've probably solved more crimes during this interview than they have in the last year," thought Charlie, eyeing the grinning detectives.

"Right," said Belly, finally, "think we've covered everything. Time to go back to the cell."

Charlie sat in his cell, staring at the bell. He would only press the bell if he wanted a cigarette or a glass of water.

"Sex tester," someone had scrawled by the bell, "press this and a cunt will appear."

"Didn't have much choice," mused Charlie, lying on the wooden bench, "once the intrusive thoughts took hold and without Colin..... what could I do?"

Charlie was taken before the custody sergeant and charged with burglaries and thefts. The remainder were to be taken into consideration.

"We will be opposing bail," said the sergeant, "on the grounds that you are likely to commit further offences. You will be taken to court in the morning."

"So what," answered Charlie, "couldn't really care."

Back in his cell, Charlie tried, unsuccessfully, to get some sleep.

"Doubt anyone will be surprised I've been nicked," he

mused, "I'm just an accident waiting to happen. Now we'll find out if adult prison is any different to young offenders."

The morning dawned with a chilly breeze and a trip to Dorking Magistrates' Court.

"You will not be granted bail," announced the magistrate, eyes front, tone level, "you will be remanded in custody for seven days."

Charlie, escorted by a young, almost boyish, jailer, returned to the court cells.

"Van won't be long, mate," said the jailer, "you'll soon be at Lewes."

"Wonder why John the jailer ain't here," thought Charlie, "this bloke looks like he should still be at school."

Lewes prison….. the old place hadn't changed. At the top of a hill, the massive stone walls surrounded the solid, old buildings. All entrances were barred and secure. The exercise yard was a rare open space within the confines.

"It seems as if I could have been here only yesterday," thought Charlie, "everything looks just as it was. Still, now I'm twenty-two so it'll be C wing."

Charlie sat in reception waiting to be taken onto the wing. Five other inmates were in the locked room. It was over an hour before a prison officer unlocked the door. They were given kit and led across the yard in the direction of C wing. He walked into the wing, desperate to remain anonymous. The prisoners were slopping-out, so he had no chance of reaching his cell without being noticed. The noise lessened as everyone tried to size up the new arrivals.

The banging of doors, the clanging on metal stairs, the jangle of keys, the shouting, the stench of stale urine…….
Charlie was back..

"We'll have some fun with you," jeered a stocky prisoner with a spider's web tattooed across his face.

"We'll see," answered Charlie, full of false bravado.

Charlie was taken to his cell.

"Hope my cellmate is alright," he thought, pushing the door, "it ain't gonna be much fun if we don't get on."

He looked at the prisoner sitting on his bed reading a magazine. A big bloke, aged around 30, heavily built, cropped black hair, battered good looks and multiple tattoos.

"Hello, mate," said Charlie, "looks like you're stuck with me."

"I'm Darren," said the prisoner, "what you done?"

"Bit of thieving," replied Charlie, "what about you?"

"Armed robbery...... couple of banks and a post office," answered Darren, "going to be a long stretch this time."

"Have you done much time?" asked Charlie.

"Too much," said Darren, "longest sentence, so far, was seven years."

"What for?" Charlie questioned.

"Street robbery," answered Darren, "held a bloke at knife-point and took his wallet and a bit of jewellery."

"What do you reckon you'll get this time?" Charlie asked.

"Solicitor reckons about twelve years. Even though I never fired it, the gun was loaded and the police found it. I'm well fucked."

"Could have been much worse," thought Charlie, "Darren ain't bad, at all. Nice bloke, even if he does look like a nutter."

"What's it like on this wing?" Charlie asked.

"It ain't that bad," answered Darren, "I just try and keep my head down and do my bird."

"Had any trouble since you've been here?"

"A geezer cut me cause he wanted my tobacco," answered Darren.

"Did you give it to him?" Charlie asked.

"No fucking chance. When he turned to leave the cell, I hit the cunt, over the head, with my chair. He ain't bothered me since. I can't let people take the piss cause I'm gonna be here for years."

"I know what you mean," thought Charlie, "with my problems, I could be here for most of my life."

Charlie sat on his bed and rolled a cigarette.

"Do you do anything during the day?" Charlie asked.

"Go to classes," answered Darren, "don't have to do anything cause I ain't convicted, but it helps to pass the time."

Inside prison or lying on a tropical beach, day follows night. Charlie sat in his cell, reading. Darren had gone to study Alfred the Great about an hour earlier.

"Slop-out," bellowed the warden, unlocking the door.

Charlie washed his plastic plates in the recess, used the

toilet and, then, walked back to his cell.

"Keep yourself to yourself," he thought, "familiarity breeds contempt."

He gazed out of the cell window, watching as convicted prisoners tended the gardens.

"Got anything for us?"

Charlie turned, sharply. An inmate, tall, athletic build, long greasy hair, untidy beard, tattooed neck, jeans and ripped leather jacket stood within a few feet. A shorter prisoner, more fat than athletic, but similarly dressed, lingered by the cell door. The door had been almost closed..... nobody wanted to be disturbed.

"Oh no," thought Charlie, "just what I didn't want."

"Where's your snout? We ain't got all day."

"It'd be much easier just to give them my fags," pondered Charlie, "I could really do without a beating."

The taller prisoner stepped forward.

"It's make your mind up time," reasoned Charlie, "give them the fags or suffer the consequences."

He looked at the prisoner.

"I just can't be taken for a prick," he decided, "as much as I'd like to avoid any trouble...... what choice have I got? Might have to spend years in prison and the tobacco is just the beginning."

"Look, mate," said Charlie, tone soft, "can't do it."

"Don't be silly," snarled the taller prisoner, "snout or we'll do ya!"

"No chance," said Charlie, tone softer, stepping backwards.

As a cigarette follows sexual intercourse, action followed the threats.

The fist smashed into Charlie's cheek. Charlie staggered backwards, the wall keeping him upright.

"Fight or flight," he thought, panicking.

Unfortunately, trapped in cell nineteen, flight wasn't an option.

He lunged forward and grabbed his attacker.

"If I just stand here," he thought, "I'm just an open target. He'll murder me."

Charlie gripped the leather jacket.It was torn, and stank.

"Hold on," he urged, "for fuck's sake..... hold on."

The prisoner struggled violently. He wanted to cause

damage and that would be much easier, and quicker, without this bald inmate hanging off him.

"Right cunt, you're dead," he snarled, shooting a glance towards the door.

Nothing was said… it didn't need to be. The look-out joined the attack. Charlie felt two sharp blows on the back of his head. He released his grip. The next flurry of punches sent him to the floor. He covered his head and curled up, praying for an end.

"All this," thought Charlie, "for a few fags."

Each kick hurt more than the one before. It seemed like minutes, but was, probably, a matter of seconds.

"What a wanker. Not worth doing a life sentence. Let's go."

The two prisoners, point proved, left the cell.

"Bastards," muttered Charlie, lying still, "hope there's no permanent damage."

After a few minutes, Charlie pulled himself, gently, onto his bed.

"I feel fucking sore," he thought, "not as much blood as you'd expect but, shit, do I ache."

The towel turned a light shade of red as Charlie wiped his face and nose.

"I ain't moving," thought Charlie, "I'm gonna just lie on this bed 'til my body stops hurting."

"Bang-up, lads," ordered the warden, slamming the door.

"Well," thought Charlie, "I've had more enjoyable slop-outs. Hope Darren is having more fun at his class."

Darren was back before lunch.

"What happened to you?" Darren asked, "you look bloody awful."

"Oh, it ain't as bad as it looks," replied Charlie, "had a bit of trouble with two geezers……….. leather jackets, jeans, scruffy long hair, tattoos……"

"Oh, what a surprise," said Darren, "Singer and Booth. What did they want?"

"Tobacco," answered Charlie.

"They're always taxing people," said Darren, "did you give it to them?"

"No," replied Charlie, feeling a lump on his head, "but it would have been easier."

"Try and forget it," said Darren, "they'll be inside for

years……. drugs, robbery, extortion, you name it."

Days passed and the bruises faded but, mentally, Charlie struggled. One slop-out, on a visit to the recess, Charlie had the pleasure of meeting Terry Percival. The prisoner walked straight into Charlie, sending his plates and cup crashing to the floor.
"Careful," said Charlie.
"Suck my dick," replied Percival.
Charlie gathered his plates and cup from the floor, stared at Percival, then went back to his cell.
"Just bumped into Percival, the wing cleaner," said Charlie to Darren, "bit of a charmer."
"Bit of a crackpot," replied Darren, "looking at murder….. think it was his best mate. Looking at life, possibly loony bin."
The following day, after lunchtime slop-out, Charlie sat in his cell trying to write a letter to Edward.
"Just can't think of anything to put," he mused.
Darren was writing to his wife.

A scream shook Charlie back into reality.
"What the fuck's that?" Charlie asked Darren.
"Don't know," replied Darren, "have a look. The flap on the door is open."
Charlie got up and went over to the door. He lowered his head and peered through the flap.
"Fucking hell," he muttered.
Terry Percival stood in the middle of the landing. One hand held a razor blade, slashing wildly at his own body. Blood dripped from both wrists and it seemed he'd slashed his own throat, too. He screamed like a madman as the razor shredded his face.
"It's Percival," said Charlie to Darren, "I think he's gone mad. Come and see."
Charlie and Darren watched as wardens surrounded the prisoner.
"There's loads of 'em", said Charlie to Darren.
"Can't be too careful, can they," replied Darren, "he's totally unstable and there's claret everywhere."
The group moved slowly along the landing.
"What do you reckon set him off?" Charlie asked.
"I ain't sure," replied Darren, "but I heard, through the

grapevine, that he got a letter from his wife telling him that she'd met someone else."

"Oh," said Charlie, watching as the group disappeared from view.

That evening, during slop-out, Charlie walked passed two wardens, covered head to toe in white protective clothing, cleaning the remains of the blood.

He had spent almost fourteen days in Lewes. Now, he was due a visit to Dorking Magistrates' Court.

John the jailer met the prison van.

"Hello Charlie," he said, "you back again?"

"'Fraid so, mate."

"Any chance of bail today?" John asked.

"No," answered Charlie, "not even going to try."

"You won't be going back to Lewes," said John, "all Surrey prisoners will be held at Highdown Prison. It's only just opened."

"Oh, right," said Charlie, "where is Highdown?"

"Near Sutton," replied John.

After a brief court appearance, an inedible lunch and a short journey in a mobile cage, Charlie had his first impressions of Highdown Prison.

"Looks okay," he pondered, "modern buildings. Very different to Lewes. Looks very secure with fences and wires everywhere. The car park in front of the walls is massive and, just down the road, only about a hundred metres or so, it looks like there's another prison. It's all surrounded by acres of trees and fields."

Charlie and his fellow prisoners were taken from the prison van and escorted to reception.

"This looks so bright and cheerful," thought Charlie, "apart from all the bars and locks, you wouldn't believe you were in a prison."

Next stop for the new inmates was a secure holding room. Three sides made of thick concrete, the fourth being a barred gate.

"Certainly no way out of here," pondered Charlie.

Each inmate was individually processed and taken to another, identical, holding room.

"Hope the screws ain't too long," thought Charlie, "just want to get on the wing."

Be careful what you wish for! Highdown's wings, or house-blocks, had a very different look to that of a Victorian jail, such as Lewes. Much smaller, with only three landings, and much cleaner.
"Not that bad," decided Charlie, "very clean, in fact. Can't even smell piss."
He was escorted to a single cell by a young officer, who was tall, slim with acne scars.
"Enjoy your stay," said Pizza Face, grinning, "may it be all you hoped for."
Charlie unpacked his few belongings and lay on the bed.
"I'm knackered," he pondered, "ain't sure why. Don't exactly do much!"
He looked at the walls, admiring the many naked ladies on display.
"Amazing what newspapers print," he thought, "still, the last bloke had good taste."
He rolled a cigarette.
"Wonder what this place will be like," he mused, "got to be better than the last shit-hole."
Charlie struggled off his bed and paced the cell. He looked out of the barred window.
"The exercise yard," he mumbled, "great view. Complete with helicopter wires to stop anyone trying to escape."
Charlie turned and paced, then turned and paced some more.
"Hope the obtrusive thoughts stay buried," he mused, "I really don't need to worry about cursing anyone."

The days passed, intrusion free. Midweek, and the door swung open. Charlie, familiar with his routine, waited with his plates.
"Alright, Ian," he said, "wonder what muck we'll get today."
Ian, an old age prisoner, thinning on top, short and round, with a well- weathered face, limped towards Charlie.
"Can't really face it," he answered.
"Not good at the moment?" Charlie asked.
"Bit worried about court," replied Ian, "spoke to my solicitor last week and he is certain I'll get off with manslaughter. Says, there's no way the murder charge will stick. But I just don't know…."

A CRY FOR EVER

"What else did he say?" Charlie enquired.
"That I've just got to tell the truth. The bloke attacked me, I grabbed the knife and, just to defend myself, stabbed him."
"You'll be fine, I'm sure," said Charlie.
"I really hope so," said Ian, "just terrified of getting life. I'm too old now... I'd never get out."
"Lunch," bellowed Pizza Face, "get a move on."
Charlie and Ian joined the queue.

The following week, during afternoon association, Charlie and a new arrival, Mike, waited for a game of pool.
Mike was almost twenty-three, tall, thin with gaunt features, untidy dark hair and was obviously a lover of body-art. He had spent much of his life in one institution or another.
"Never get fucking bail," he moaned, "only here for two non-dwellings."
"Did you try for bail?" asked Charlie.
"Yeah," answered Mike, "but they said I'd keep offending, and put me in here."
"What do you reckon you'll get?" Charlie asked.
"Solicitor reckons a couple of years, this time," answered Mike, "eighteen months, if I'm lucky."

Charlie and Mike watched a couple of feeble shots on the green baize.
"What do you reckon on the food?" Mike asked.
"It ain't all that great, is it?" answered Charlie.
"Go and have a look at the suggestions book," said Mike, "I wrote a comment after my first meal."
"Okay," answered Charlie.
He walked towards the table where the book, filled with untidy scrawl, was kept. A prisoner, who couldn't have been older than twenty-one, scowled as he studied the book. Charlie tried to see the page, hoping to read Mike's comment. He moved closer to the young man as he struggled to decipher the uneducated ramblings.
"Why don't you fuck off, you bald cunt," shouted the inmate, turning his scowling face and pointing a tattooed finger.
"Shit," panicked Charlie, "what the fuck......."
Charlie backed away from the stocky, heavily tattooed prisoner without a hint of resistance. He went straight to his cell and threw himself onto the bed.

"Shit," he muttered, "what the fuck did he do that for? He made me look a complete wanker in front of the whole wing. I'd rather just forget it but..... I can't. If I just leave it....... well, I just can't."

He lay on the bed. It seemed like ages until the door slamming signalled the end of association.

"Just got to do something," he muttered.

Charlie looked at his radio or, more importantly, the PP9 battery connected to it.

"Lots of people used those batteries when I was a young offender," he thought, "a lump of solid metal...... perfect."

He disconnected the battery, then took a sock from his cupboard..... a lethal weapon!

"Don't reckon I'll have the bottle," he thought, swinging the battery inside the sock, "I just won't be able to do it."

He paced the cell, shaking with anticipation, an emotional wreck.

"Got to do it," he muttered, "with the intrusions so fucking bad might be in prison for years. Can't be taken for a prick all the time."

"Association," yelled the warden, unlocking the cell.

Charlie, legs unsteady, hurried towards Mike's cell.

"No point in hanging about," he decided, "if I don't do it now, my bottle will go."

Mike was sitting at his table, pen in hand, trying to finish his reception letter.

"Mike," said Charlie, "could you do me a favour?"

"Sure," answered Mike, "as long as it's nothing sexual."

"Just come with me," said Charlie.

Charlie, legs even more unsteady, crossed the landing with Mike a few paces behind. Cell fourteen held a young prisoner known for temper tantrums.

"Just stay outside and watch for screws," said Charlie.

Mike nodded his agreement.

"Perfect," reasoned Charlie, "not only can Mike keep look-out, but he'll be a witness. He'll know I'm not a complete pushover and, in prison, when one person knows something, it doesn't take long before jungle drums are beating. And, if things go wrong and I'm getting a beating, hopefully, he'll help me."

Charlie walked into cell fourteen, the battery and sock

concealed inside his clothing. The young inmate lay on his bed, scowling at the ceiling.

"I could just walk out and forget it," panicked Charlie.

The prisoner sat upright, still scowling.

"No turning back," decided Charlie: fight not flight.

"What do you want?" growled the prisoner.

"Not much," answered Charlie, "just an apology. And I ain't leaving 'til I get one."

Charlie really hoped that he would have no use for the battery in his sock, still hidden inside his clothes, but kept it readily available.

"Surely," thought Charlie, "if he was going to attack me, he'd have done it by now."

The young prisoner glanced at the door but stayed seated.

"This might be okay," thought Charlie, "might be able to leave here with my pride intact, without having to do anything."

"For fuck's sake," said the inmate, "you were leaning over while I was trying to write. You invaded my space. You were out of order."

"Okay," said Charlie, prepared to appease, "sorry for leaning over."

The young man fidgeted, tattooed hand running through his dark, greasy mop of hair.

"This has got to be it," decided Charlie, "if I don't lash him in a minute then I'm going to look more of a tosser than I did before."

"Okay", conceded the prisoner, "I'm sorry about what happened. Happy now?"

"Yeah," replied Charlie, "suppose I am."

He turned and left. Mike followed his friend back to his cell.

"Sweet, mate," said Mike, "he was all mouth with nothing else."

"Yeah," answered Charlie, "glad to get it sorted."

Charlie and Mike sat in Lee's cell just before evening bang-up.

"Only ten minutes," said Charlie, "and that'll be another day done."

"Couldn't really care," replied Lee, "I'll be out soon, only got three months for driving on a ban."

"Do you reckon you'll ever come back?" Mike asked.

"Do you enjoy a blow-job?" Lee laughed, "I'm lucky only to

be here for driving while banned. Could be much worse. The week before I went to court, I was questioned about other things, much worse things."

"Like what?" Mike asked.

"A lad was glassed in a fight outside a club," said Lee, "lost the sight in one eye and had seventeen stitches."

"Oh," said Mike, "was it you?"

"Who knows," replied Lee.

"Anything else?" Mike asked.

"Me and a mate were stopped in a stolen car with gear from four or five robberies," answered Lee, "but my mate told the coppers he'd just given me a ride and it was nothing to do with me. It's important to have good mates."

Lee stood up to pour a cup of water.

"He's so short," thought Charlie, "probably not much more than five feet. Reckon he's like a terrier…. just keeps going at you 'til you can't take no more."

"Bang-up," bellowed Pizza Face, from the landing, "back to your own cells."

The door clanged open. Another day, same as the one before. Charlie struggled out of bed. First job….. roll a fag.

"Morning, Chaz," said Lee, strolling into the cell, "get your hand off your cock, it's eight o'clock."

"Morning, mate," yawned Charlie, inhaling deeply.

"Not stopping," said Lee, " nearly time for breakfast. It's cornflakes today."

Charlie scrambled into his clothes, then stumbled to the back of the breakfast queue.

"Seems to be more people by the day," he thought, "police must be busy."

The conveyor belt moved quickly. Charlie reached the front of the queue and held out a blue, plastic plate. The server, a six-foot, eighteen stone armed robber, slapped a grisly piece of bacon on his plate.

"Thanks mate," said Charlie.

"That's okay."

"You lousy wanker!" Charlie flinched at the intrusion.

He collected the rest of his food, eyes watching the armed robber.

"He ain't looking at me," reasoned Charlie, "I definitely didn't say anything. It was a bloody thought but I didn't say it aloud."

A CRY FOR EVER

Charlie filled his cup with boiling water, shot a last look at the armed robber, and walked to his cell.

"Nothing happened," he pondered, "it was all in my fucking screwed-up head."

"You can't be one hundred per cent on that, can you?"

He couldn't face breakfast. He lit a roll-up instead.

"I know," he decided, "I'll speak to the bloke at lunch. It's always the same prisoners serving the grub. He'll remember me if I've said anything bad. Not to mention, he'd probably break every bone in my body."

Most of the morning, Charlie spent pacing the cell. He wasn't hungry; his stomach was in knots, but he needed to know.

"Just got to clear this worry," mused Charlie, "can't function 'til I know it's okay."

"Lunch," yelled Pizza Face at last, unlocking the door.

"Does that cunt ever go home?" he thought, "either his wife is frigid or he needs extra cash."

Charlie grabbed his plates and cup, left the cell and headed for the front of the queue.

"Just want to get this over with," he thought.

His heart pounded, his mouth was dry and the plastic plates and cup shook in his hands as he walked towards the servers.

"Good," he thought, "the same bloke is serving. I hoped he would be."

He walked closer, praying his legs would hold him.

"Oh shit," he mumbled, "he's serving the liver. If there's one thing I hate, it's liver."

However, today, the liver could taste like used spunk.

"Needs must," he reasoned.

Charlie held out his plate, trying to disguise his unsteady hand.

"Alright, mate," stammered Charlie, " having a good day?"

"Not that bad," replied armed robber, placing the liver on Charlie's plate, "that's a good piece."

"Thanks," said Charlie, "I'll enjoy that."

He scuttled back to his cell. He was walking on air. England were going to win the World Cup and he'd be trapped in a lift with a gorgeous nymphomaniac.

"Great," he thought, "a normal response. Reckon that'll clear the worry."

The delighted prisoner threw his slice of liver in the waste-bin.

Evening association. It was nearly the weekend, and Charlie stood beside the pool table chatting to Ian.

"Who do you knock about with on the outside?" Ian asked.

"Well," answered Charlie, "I had a best mate - Colin. We used to do most things together...... pull birds, and all that. Don't ask me why but he topped himself. Knew he was a bit pissed off but didn't expect anything like that."

"That's heavy," said Ian, "what shit."

Ian took his tobacco from his pocket.

"Really wish I could stop smoking," he said, "have to see the nurse, once a week, cause of bad circulation in my legs."

He rolled a cigarette.

"How long ago did Colin kill himself?" Ian asked.

"Not long before I came in here," replied Charlie, "I found it so difficult to manage without him. Life wasn't really worth it."

"What do you want to do with your life?" Ian asked.

"I ain't really got a plan," answered Charlie, "probably keep coming to places like this."

"What a waste," said Ian.

"I know what you mean," answered Charlie.

"I've spent over twenty years in custody," said Ian, "and now, when I look back, I wonder why I've wasted my life. The first time I went to Borstal was at sixteen. I'd nicked a couple of cars and burgled a shop. All my mates came to court with me and I felt a right hero. When I came out, lots of my mates were busy with other things....... girls, work..... loads of stuff."

"How long did you do?" Charlie asked.

"Twenty-one months," answered Ian.

"Long time for a couple of cars and a shop," said Charlie.

"Yeah," replied Ian, " and it didn't do any good. I was only out for about six months before I was sent back. This time, only a couple of mates came to court. I didn't realise it, but, gradually, I was losing touch with the outside."

"Yeah, I see," said Charlie.

"I done another twenty-three months and, when I got out, I had nobody."

"What did you do?" Charlie asked.

"In my mind," said Ian, "I didn't have a choice. I carried on thieving and, before long, I was serving five years in prison."

"Oh," said Charlie.

"I'd give anything to have my time again. Would find myself a reason to stay away from crime and prison."

"I know what you mean," said Charlie.

"You see," continued Ian, "everyone wants to be needed. Colin was needed but just didn't realise how much. Would he have been so depressed if he knew what he meant to people?"

"I ain't sure," said Charlie, "maybe not."

"Linda, your girlfriend. Is it serious?"

"Not really," replied Charlie, "bit of a laugh."

"Thought you had a baby," said Ian.

"We do," answered Charlie, "love the baby but, as for Linda......."

"Well," said Ian, "your baby needs you. She won't judge your past. Love her and she'll save you. Love is stronger than desire. I reckon you've robbed your last shop."

"Maybe....," muttered Charlie.

"The table is free," said Ian, "want a thrashing?"

"Two roll-ups says that won't happen."

Association ended, prisoners were banged up, daytime staff went home to moaning wives, and the nightshift came on duty.

Charlie lay in his cell, staring at the ceiling. Voices echoed around the prison.

"Window warriors are on form tonight," thought Charlie, listening.

"If you killed me, then you'd be doing me a favour," screeched a voice, "I've got Parkinson's so I'll be dead soon anyway. And you'll do a life sentence."

"If I killed you," bellowed the reply, "I'd be doing everyone a favour."

Charlie put his head under the pillow.

"I suppose I could be a good father," he pondered, "don't want much to do with Linda but I'd love to play a part in Charlotte's life."

"My missus gives great head," a voice yelled across the exercise yard.

"I know," boomed the reply.

"Shit," muttered Charlie, "how am I going to sleep?"

He clambered off the bed and sat at his table.

"Might as well have a fag," he decided.

He rolled a skinny cigarette and poured a cup of water.

"Charlotte didn't ask to be born," he pondered, "so I must make sure that she has a good life. She looked so innocent at the hospital, she needs me more than anyone."

The voices continued:

"I don't care which screws are about, tomorrow I'm gonna fucking do ya."

"Try it, you fucker."

"Charming," thought Charlie, "what a lovely class of resident."

He finished his cigarette, cleaned his teeth and flopped onto the bed.

"I'll write to my solicitor in the morning and tell him to try for bail," he thought, "must start as I mean to go on. Ain't much use to Charlotte in here."

He pulled the green blanket over his head. Despite voices from all directions, he eventually fell asleep.

"Morning," yelled Pizza Face, opening the cell.

"Not him again," thought Charlie, hopping out of bed.

He collected his breakfast, ate what he could and settled down to write a letter to Mr Gordon, his solicitor.

He ended, "…and to help with my application for bail, please could you contact Dr. King and ask for a psychiatric report. I feel this would be to my advantage and should help the magistrates come to a decision in my favour. Look forward to seeing you on Tuesday.

Best wishes, Charlie Lloyd."

Monday afternoon, dry and bright, and Charlie fancied a stroll in the exercise yard. The inmates walked, anti-clockwise, around the perimeter of the wall. Most were in pairs, some in groups of three or four. Charlie walked with Martin, a young man whose life had been totally destroyed by drugs.

"Are you on remand?" Charlie asked.

"Yeah," replied Martin.

"What for? Charlie enquired.

"Well," answered Martin, "I was caught for shoplifting and the bastards found a load of heroin."

"How long do you reckon you'll get?" Charlie asked.

"Really ain't sure," replied Martin.

They must have walked round the yard over fifty times.

"Look," said Martin, pointing.

A skinhead, face and neck covered in tattoos, was hitting another prisoner, who was cowering on the floor. The wardens strolled, casually, towards the beating. You'd have been excused for thinking they were strolling along a beach on a summer's evening.

"The screws ain't exactly rushing," said Charlie.

"Probably ain't bothered," replied Martin, "from what I heard the bloke on the ground is a bit of a weirdo. They probably reckon he deserves it."

The officers, finally, separated the pair and took them away. Two wardens dragged the skinhead to the block and another took the injured prisoner for a medical check-up. Two officers remained on exercise duty, looking thoroughly fed up.

"End of exercise. Bang-up, lads," yelled the warden.

Martin and Charlie followed the stream of inmates onto the wing.

"See you later, Martin," said Charlie.

"Yeah, at tea," replied Martin.

"You junkie slag."

Charlie sat in his cell with his head in his hands.

"Fuck," he panicked, "did I say anything?"

He stared at the bars across his window.

"The bars keep me here," he pondered, "but, even when they let me out, will I ever be free?"

He picked up his book, but the words might as well have been written in Chinese.

"I just can't fucking concentrate," he thought, "I'll have to check with Martin, so I can stop worrying"

 But at tea, there was no sign of Martin. Charlie collected his meal but didn't even try it.

"Association," shouted the warden, opening the door.

Charlie hurried onto the landing. Still no Martin!

Charlie walked over to Ian.

"Have you seen Martin since tea?" Charlie asked, "short chap, greasy hair…… cell thirty-one."

"I heard he'd been taken down the block," replied Ian, "not sure if it's true, but I think they found some drugs in his cell."

"Shit," muttered Charlie.

"Sure he'll be fine," said Ian, "don't worry."

Association passed in a whirl. Afterwards, Charlie sat on his bed staring at a naked lady with a massive chest.

"Bollocks," he thought, "really wanted to check with Martin, to see if I said anything. I'll be taken to court before he's unlocked for breakfast, but, if he's back from the block, I could shout through his door."

He lay under his covers.

"Got to try and sleep," he thought, "sooner I sleep, sooner I can stop worrying. This reminds me of being a kid on Christmas Eve: can't sleep 'cause I'm so desperate for the next day."

Charlie fidgeted, then turned over his pillow. The other side was always cooler. The anxiety lessened, then, without warning, the worry came back.

"It's like a bad dream," thought Charlie, "you're running, desperately trying to get away from the bogey man but, however fast you run, wherever you hide, he always finds you. You just can't get rid of him. At least, not 'til you wake up. Waking up means I'll being able to check it all out and stop worrying. If you don't wake up…… who knows how long the anxiety will last?"

Charlie must have fallen asleep, as he was woken by the jangle of keys and the door being unlocked.

"Lloyd," said the warden, "you're in court today. Get your stuff together and wait at the gate."

"Okay, guv," said Charlie.

He dressed, grabbed his belongings and hurried out of the cell. He headed straight for cell thirty-one.

"Don't feel so shit, this morning," he thought, "but it'll be nice to check out that it's all okay."

The landings were almost empty, as only the prisoners in court that day had been unlocked.

Charlie peered through the flap on cell thirty-one.

"Pucker," he murmured, "Martin's back from the block."

The covers moved as Martin stirred in his sleep.

"Martin," Charlie whispered, "come to your door."

No response.

"Martin," said Charlie, a little louder, "wake up."

Still no reaction.

"Martin," said Charlie, almost shouting, "for fuck's sake, get up."

The covers moved and a mop of messy hair lifted off the pillow. A pair of eyes squinted in the darkness, trying to identify the nuisance at the door.

"Martin, it's me, Charlie," he said, "come over here."

"What's the matter?" Martin muttered, stumbling to the door.

"Nothing to worry about," whispered Charlie, "I'm in court today and might get a bit of bail. Just wanted to wish you all the best and give you some burn. I've got quite a bit and, if all goes to plan, I won't need it."

Charlie pushed a tobacco pouch under the door.

"Thanks," said Martin, "be lucky."

"You too," answered Charlie, "better go."

Charlie turned and headed down the landing to join the other prisoners at the gate.

"Worry over," he thought, "now I can concentrate on bail."

On a natural high, he arrived at Dorking Magistrates' Court.

"Double bubble, today," he pondered, "cleared a worry and got a chance of bail."

"Hello, Charlie," said John the jailer, "glad to be back? I'll take you to your cell."

"Thanks, guv," replied Charlie, "going for bail today."

Charlie sat in the cell underneath the courts, drinking a cup of tea and smoking a roll-up.

"Can't wait to see Charlotte," he mused, "hope I can get things right. Hope the bloody intrusions don't make things so bad that I just come straight back."

John opened the door and handed Charlie some lunch.

"Your mum is in court," said John, "she's been here all day."

"Thanks guv," said Charlie.

Charlie ate his lunch, drank his tea, smoked a roll-up and paced the cell.

"Hope I get bail," he pondered, "my life starts today."

It wasn't long before John unlocked the door.

"Your solicitor is here, Charlie," he said.

Mr. Gordon, who Charlie thought of as 'Flash', walked into the cell, glanced briefly at his papers, then cleared his throat.

"Well," he said, "we are ready to apply for bail. I've spoken to Dr. King and we've managed to put together a psychiatric report."

"What are the chances of bail?" Charlie asked.

"Well," answered Flash, "the psychiatric report will be a great help. I will do my best. Let's just wait and see."

Flash left the cell. Then John locked the door, and Charlie was left pacing up and down.

It wasn't long, about fifteen minutes, before the door swung open.

"You're on, Charlie," said John, "best of luck. Hope I don't see you back in this cell. Except when you collect your property, of course."

Charlie stood in the dock. He smiled at his mother in the gallery, then faced the front.

The prosecution began to outline their case.

"...... this young man has many convictions for dishonesty and, we believe, if released would continue to commit offences....."

Charlie shuffled, nervously, in the dock.

"This bloke would make a monk look like a sex addict," thought Charlie, "I'm going back to Highdown."

The prosecutor droned on .... and on.

"He obviously didn't get his pecker felt last night," pondered Charlie, " and now he wants to make sure that I'm in the same boat."

Finally, the prosecutor, beads of perspiration glistening on his brow, sat down.

"Thank fuck," thought Charlie, "what a stirrer."

Mr. Gordon scrambled to his feet.

"I believe," began Flash, "this is a chance for my client to change direction in his life. As you can see from the psychiatric report, my client has a treatable condition. Prison will only to serve to aggravate his condition. In the community he can be treated. In his own misdirected way, my client has tried to protect the community from himself. He has a baby daughter and really feels a responsibility towards her. His mother, in court today, takes a keen interest in his welfare......"

"Bloody good," thought Charlie, "I'm sure the female magistrate is trying not to cry."

"So," concluded Flash, "as my client will happily visit Dr. King as an outpatient, I would urge that bail should be granted."

"We shall retire," announced the presiding magistrate, adjusting his glasses.

A CRY FOR EVER

Charlie sat in the dock, eyes fixed on the floor.
"Reckon I'll get bail," he pondered, "Flash was shit hot."

It seemed an eternity, but was probably only a few minutes, until the magistrates shuffled back into the courtroom.
"We are granting bail......." began Bins
"Thank fuck," thought Charlie.
".........and failure to surrender is viewed most seriously." concluded Bins.
Charlie grinned at his mother and left the dock.
"I've got to make the most of this chance," he thought, "just as long as the intrusions don't fuck it for me."
Charlie grabbed his belongings from the cell and shook John's hand.
"Thanks guv," said Charlie, "be lucky."
"You too, mate," replied John
"He's far too nice to be a screw," thought Charlie.

Charlie walked to the waiting area and found Mr. Gordon with his mother.
"Thank-you, Mr. Gordon," said Charlie, "really grateful."
Charlie and his mother left the court and walked the short distance to the car-park.
"So far, so good," thought Charlie, "no old women, no intrusions........ could things be any better?"

Chapter 4

Charlie opened the door and slumped into the car.

"No old women," he thought, checking his surroundings, "and no worries."

His mother started the car, checked and pulled away.

"I'm going to live at Linda's," said Charlie, "and try and get to know Charlotte."

"If that's what you want," sighed Hazel, "then give it a go."

"Don't you reckon it's for the best?" Charlie asked.

"I hope it works for you," replied his mother, "and if it doesn't you can always come home."

"Back at last," said Charlie, staring at the bungalow.

He clambered out of the car and went inside.

"First job," he decided, "a proper cup of coffee and a fag."

He sat at the kitchen table, drinking and smoking.

"Luxury," he pondered, "this has been worth the wait."

"How have you been?" Hazel asked.

"Oh, not too bad," answered Charlie, "but, now I really want to be involved with Charlotte."

Charlie finished his coffee, stubbed his roll-up in the ashtray and stood up.

"Just going to have a bath," he said, " and then I'll phone Linda."

He soaked in the steaming tub.

"Nice to have some privacy," he mused, glancing at the locked door, "and not worry who is going to come in."

He splashed his face, enjoying the sensation.

"Wonder if I'll ever go back to prison," he pondered, "I suppose that depends on the intrusions. At the moment I'm determined to stay out, and make a go of it with Charlotte, but if the intrusions get really bad then….. fuck knows."

Charlie, washed, dried and dressed, went to phone Linda.

"Hello Linda," he said, "got bail today."

"Lucky you," she said, "was it ok?"

"Pretty normal," answered Charlie.

"Will you be round later?" Linda asked.

"Well," begun Charlie, "I've been thinking and….. um….. if it's ok with you, I'd like to live with you and Charlotte."

Silence.

"I really want to play a part in Charlotte's life," continued

A CRY FOR EVER

Charlie. "Nothing heavy, no commitment. I'll sleep in the spare room and take care of Charlotte."

Silence.

"It'll give you a break," offered Charlie, "I mean, it must be so difficult with three children."

"So," answered Linda, "you want to live with Charlotte. Couldn't give a flying fuck about me, Becky or Alan but....... you want to live here."

"I wouldn't put it like that," replied Charlie, "but now that we've got Charlotte, I would like to be more involved."

"Okay Charlie," said Linda, "do what you like."

"I'll be round this evening," answered Charlie.

He sat at the kitchen table, roll-up in one hand and coffee mug in the other.

"I hope I'm doing the right thing," he pondered, "I suppose this is the best chance of forming a bond with Charlotte. And, to be honest, I've only got to sleep at Linda's house; during the day I can come back here."

Later, grasping a bag of clean clothes, he knocked on Linda's front door.

"Front garden is a bit overgrown," he thought, "could go to the shop and never be seen again."

"Hello," said Linda, opening the door, "you came then."

"Looks like it," replied Charlie, "and I've got everything I'll need for a while."

Charlie walked into the lounge. Becky and Alan were drawing on the walls.

"Hello," he mumbled.

Charlotte was asleep on the sofa.

"Amazing," he thought, "how she can sleep with all this noise?"

Linda sat on a chair in front of the television.

"Don't fucking do that," she yelled, staring at Becky and Alan.

They hesitated, then decided it would be safer to colour on paper.

"I hope I can cope with this," thought Charlie, "I really do."

Charlie headed for the stairs.

"Just going to sort out the spare room," he muttered to Linda, "won't be long."

Charlie opened the door and studied his new 'home'.

"Bit of a shit-hole," he thought, "could do with a good clean, new carpet, bit of fresh paint.........."

He unpacked his clobber, making sure his medication was out of the reach of any wandering hands.

"Still," he pondered, " won't be here that much."

He walked into Linda's room. Charlotte's cot stood between the dirty bed and battered wardrobe.

"I won't give her the chance to say no," decided Charlie, I'll put the cot in my room."

Charlie grinned as he placed the cot at the end of his bed.

He walked into the lounge. Alan yanked Becky's hair. Becky cried and Linda swore.

"I've put the cot in my room," said Charlie, "at least you should get a good sleep."

"Whatever, Charlie," Linda snapped, "do what the fuck you want."

A hungry baby's cry is impossible to ignore. Charlie dragged himself from his pit.

"Four o'clock in the morning," he murmured, squinting at the bedside clock.

He struggled to the kitchen, warmed a bottle and returned to the screaming infant.

"Here you are, Tiger," he whispered, "reckon this is what you want."

Another night, another feed.

"Ain't sure if it gets any easier," thought Charlie, "suppose you get used to being dragged out of bed at all hours."

Quarter to five and the bottle was empty. Charlie lay Charlotte in her cot and snuggled under his covers.

"She should be okay 'til morning," he decided, "I'll just get as much sleep as I can."

A Tuesday morning, sunny but chilly.

"Mummy has gone shopping," said Charlie, fastening Charlotte's coat, "shall we go for a walk round the park?"

He strapped Charlotte into her pushchair, covered her with a blanket and left the house.

He checked his surroundings.

"No old women," he thought, "come on, it's going to be fine."

Ten minutes, no old women, and Charlie stood at the edge of the field.

"Everything okay," he decided, " a couple of toddlers, carefully watched by their mum, on the play area and a

50

middle-aged man walking his dog."

Charlie went round the field, enjoying a sense of freedom.

"It's nice here," he said to Charlotte, "peaceful. Nothing to disturb you."

A bench, covered in graffiti, stood on the far side of the park.

"Let's sit down," said Charlie, "it's not that cold."

Charlie sat on the bench and Charlotte, snug in her pushchair, faced him.

"I used to walk everywhere with Colin," said Charlie, "I hated going out alone cause I wasn't very well, so he always came with me. Wish you could have met him. He died. Was really sad and didn't want to be here. I always wonder....... if he could of just hung on............ surely, life would have got better."

Charlotte yawned and rubbed her eyes.

"Okay," said Charlie, "I'll just have a quick fag and we'll head home."

Charlie took his tobacco out of his pocket. He glanced at the play area; it was empty. He looked in the opposite direction. An elderly lady with a Yorkshire Terrier on a lead couldn't have been further than ten yards from the bench.

"Oh no," panicked Charlie, "I don't believe it. She's heading straight for the bench."

Charlie, heart racing, replaced his tobacco and gripped the pushchair with both hands.

"Mustn't worry," he thought, "just going to keep my hands on the pushchair."

The lady, grey hair, glasses and slightly hunched, stood by the pushchair.

"May I have a look at your baby ," she asked, smiling sweetly.

"Yeah, 'course," replied Charlie, clinging to the pushchair.

"She's lovely," said the lady, "you must be so proud."

"Thank-you," replied Charlie.

Charlie's hands were starting to ache.

"Just got to hang on," he prayed, "mustn't worry. Must concentrate on what I'm doing."

Charlie looked at his hands, just to make sure they hadn't moved.

"Okay, so far," he thought, "she'll go in a minute. Not much longer."

"Is she good at night?" asked the lady.

"Er……. yeah," answered Charlie, trying to focus, "only wakes once or twice."

"Well, I'd better be going," said the lady, "lovely to meet you both."

"Did I hit her?" The intrusion grabbed its final opportunity.

Charlie stared at the elderly lady. She showed no sign of distress. Then, he looked at his hands. His fingers were still tightly wrapped round the pushchair's handle.

"Bye," said the woman, gently pulling the dog's lead, "come on, Joey."

The lady and Joey moved slowly away from the bench.

Charlie put his head in his hands.

"Shit," he thought, "is she ok? Did I hurt her?"

He felt anxious. Replaying the meeting in his mind did little to comfort him. He watched the lady and her dog crossing the park. As he watched, his anxiety lowered, but only slightly.

"Got to check she's okay," decided Charlie, "just have to know that I didn't do anything to hurt her."

He stood up and took hold of the pushchair.

"Come on, Tiger," he said, "this won't take a minute."

He followed the lady, carefully pacing himself. Quick enough to catch her before she reached the car park, but not too quickly, as he certainly didn't want to cause alarm.

"I would bet my left nipple that I didn't hurt her," thought Charlie, "but I still have to check."

With the pushchair, he drew alongside the lady and her dog.

"I'll leave a small gap between us," he thought, "have to be able to hear her but not startle her. And, whatever happens, I'll make sure there's nothing to worry about; I don't want her to get another scare."

Joey stopped and sniffed a patch of grass, seemingly fascinated.

"Hurry up, Joey," said the lady, tugging gently on the lead, "this walk has taken ages."

"Hope it doesn't rain," said Charlie, glancing at the woman, "I didn't hear the forecast."

"I'm sure it won't," she replied, with a smile, "it's cold, but I really think it'll stay dry."

"Bingo," thought Charlie, edging away from the lady and her dog, "getting rid of a worry……. it's better than sex."

Charlie turned away from the lady and hurried across the

park.
"Goodbye," he called, "take care."

It was a Thursday evening. Charlie and Charlotte sat in their room as the rain lashed against the window and the wind howled in the trees. Charlie could hear Linda, Becky and Alan downstairs.
"What the fuck did you do that for?" Linda yelled.
"He hit me first," wailed Becky.
"Oh, shut up, the pair of you," shouted Linda.
"Let's have some music, Tiger," said Charlie, going to his cupboard, "I'll just choose a tape."
He opened the cupboard door.
"Oh no," he muttered, "I had twelve tapes in here. Eleven of them have gone and this one is ruined, snapped in half."
It didn't need a genius to realise what had happened. A quick look in Becky's room revealed most of the missing tapes. Most of them had been broken into small pieces.
"Bollocks," cursed Charlie, "that's every tape .... fucked."
He walked to the top of the stairs.
"Linda," he called, "could I have a word?"
"What's the matter now?" Linda asked, climbing the stairs.
"Becky and Alan have ruined my tapes. Could you ask them not to go in my room?"
"You tell them," snapped Linda, "why the fuck are you having a go at me?"
"I was just asking you to tell them," said Charlie, "that's all."
"Oh, fuck off," answered Linda, "I don't need this shit."

Charlie lay in bed later that night, staring into the darkness. Charlotte lay in her cot, sleeping peacefully.
"This ain't no good," he pondered,"I can't stand living here. I feel so miserable and that's no good for Charlotte. In a perfect world, I'd live with Charlotte but....... not here. I have to get away and, then, I'll get things sorted."
Decision made. In the morning, he would tell Linda.

The following day, about eight o'clock, he walked into the kitchen. Linda was buttering a slice of bread.
"Look," said Charlie, "this ain't working. I'm leaving."
"Okay," replied Linda, staring at the bread, "but you ain't taking Charlotte with you."
"Okay," said Charlie, without emotion, "I still reckon it's best

for everyone."

He walked into the lounge. Charlotte lay on her mat, unaware of the chaos all around.

"Bye, Tiger," said Charlie, "I'll get things sorted. Soon."

But minutes became hours, hours became days, days became weeks. Charlie sat at the kitchen table at home, coffee cup in one hand, roll-up in the other. Some things never change!

"Got to get things sorted," he pondered, "I ain't seen Charlotte for weeks. This can't go on."

He rolled himself another cigarette.

"And I'm in court in a couple of weeks. Could get put away. Have to get things organised by then."

He walked into the lounge. A video lay on the coffee table.

"Wonder what this is," he thought, picking up the tape, "Hazel must have watched it last night."

"Kramer versus Kramer," he read, "a story about a desperate custody battle for a young child."

"Sounds topical," mused Charlie, "I'll give it a go. Nothing else to do."

Charlie started the tape. Before long he was hooked on the moving story. Two parents who would do anything to care for their child.

"That's it," decided Charlie, "I'm going round Linda's tomorrow. Whatever happens, I'm going to see Charlotte."

Charlie struggled from his pit around nine o'clock. Two coffees and three roll-ups later, he began the twenty minute stroll to Linda's house.

He walked down the hill. The morning was cold but dry.

"Hope things go okay," he mused, "what will I do if she tells me to fuck off?"

He crossed the road, turned the corner and passed the secondary school. A figure approached in the distance. He walked on, heading towards the lone pedestrian.

"Oh fuck," he muttered, close enough to see, "just my luck."

The lady, handbag in one hand, walking stick in the other, was seventy-five if she was a day.

"Really don't want to get worried," panicked Charlie.

He crossed to the other side of the road.

"Bit risky," he thought, "as there ain't no pavement. Still, needs must!"

54

A CRY FOR EVER

He walked along the road. He kept a close eye on the elderly lady, making sure that she stayed on her side of the road.

"Can't have her straying across the road," he thought, "then I might worry that I've hit her."

Charlie watched as she limped along the pavement.

"You old fucker!" Where had the intrusion come from?

He covered his mouth with his hand. He watched intently as the lady struggled on.

"Look," he reasoned, "as far as she's concerned you don't exist. You definitely didn't shout anything offensive at her. The thought entered your head but you didn't say anything aloud. It's similar to worries about hitting elderly woman - you always have to check that you've never acted on the intrusive ideas. And, let's be honest, you never have."

The lady rummaged in her handbag, completely oblivious to the anxiety she'd provoked.

Charlie stood at the side of the road, summoning the strength to progress.

"She's fine," he insisted, "you never said anything. No worries!"

The remainder of his journey was uneventful - free from the dangers presented by elderly females!

Charlie rapped on Linda's door.

"Hope she's in a good mood," he pondered, "still got to try. If you don't ask, you don't get."

The door opened.

"Oh, it's you," said Linda, "what do you want?"

"I've come to see Charlotte," answered Charlie.

"I never stopped you from seeing her," said Linda, "you were the one who fucked off."

"I know," agreed Charlie, "had to get my head sorted."

"Well, okay," said Linda, "I could use a bit of help."

"Right," said Charlie, "it's totally your choice, but I'd love to share her care. How about a week with you and then a week with me?"

"I ain't sure," answered Linda.

"You must be so busy with Becky and Alan," noted Charlie, "wouldn't it give you a bit of space?"

"A week with you and then a week with me," said Linda, "it's just − she'll get so confused."

"But," continued Charlie, "it's so important that she sees both of us."

"True," said Linda, "and the three of 'em ain't easy."

"Okay then," said Charlie, "what if I had her during the week and you looked after her at weekends?"

"Um............" Linda hesitated.

"If you ever want to see her during the week," continued Charlie, "I'll bring her straight round."

"I don't know," said Linda.

"And," said Charlie, "legally, you'll still have full custody. So, if you're not happy, you can always take her back."

"Okay," agreed Linda, "we'll give it a try."

Charlie ran home. He grabbed the phone and dialled.

"Hello, Richard," he said, " are you free for a couple of hours? Need to move some of Charlotte's gear to my house."

"Okay," replied Richard, "I'll collect you in about half an hour and we'll go to Linda's."

Bottle steriliser, clothes, nappies, baby milk and a couple of Charlotte's favourite toys fitted neatly into Richard's van.

"Good job that we don't need a cot," said Charlie, "I couldn't believe it when Lucy brought one home. Now, I'm glad she did."

Charlie strapped Charlotte into the pushchair.

"See you back at my house," he said to Richard, "I won't be too long."

Charlotte settled in quickly. Lucy was a great help, especially at night. During the day, the local park was a only a ten minute stroll away − very convenient when it was dry.

One rainy Thursday, mid-morning, Charlie and Charlotte sat in the lounge, watching Jungle Book on video.

"I really enjoy looking after Tiger," pondered Charlie, looking at her propped on the sofa, staring at the television, "it gives me a purpose. A reason to resist the intrusions. A reason to resist the temptation to go back to prison if the intrusions do manage to make my life a misery."

The rain splashed against the window. No chance of a visit to the park.

"Only a few days 'til court," mused Charlie, "pray I don't get put away. How would I cope without Tiger?"

Monday morning, clear and bright. The world would have

been a beautiful place if there hadn't been the small matter of a pending court case.

Charlie and Charlotte sat in Hazel's car. First stop…. Linda's house. She would be taking care of Charlotte while Charlie's fate was decided. Charlotte looked thrilled to see her mother.

"She doesn't need to worry about anything," thought Charlie, "as long as she has the basics, where's the problem?"

Charlie gave Linda some of Charlotte's belongings.

"Bye, Tiger," he said, "I'll see you this evening. I promise."

Charlie and his mother drove the twenty minute journey to Dorking Magistrates' Court."

"I hope that I ain't made a promise I can't keep," pondered Charlie, "that would be a terrible thing to do to a child."

He answered his bail, then returned to the waiting room to sit with Hazel until his case was called.

"If I get away with this," he pondered, "I'll never put myself in this position again. Charlotte comes first."

"Lloyd. Court 1."

"Here we go again," he thought, following the usher to the front of the courtroom, "time for reckoning."

Charlie stood nervously, staring at the three magistrates. Two men and a lady. The man, to the left, looked middle-aged with silver hair and glasses. He had a very long, narrow face and constantly frowned.

"Pin-head," decided Charlie, watching the man, "what a miserable looking fucker."

The main man, in the middle, was, putting it politely, well covered. Late forties, brown hair, chubby face and forced smile.

"Lard-boy," thought Charlie, "now we know why the bakery didn't have any pies."

The only lady on the bench, was immaculately presented, late thirties, long blonde hair, attractive facially and, although sitting, appeared nicely formed.

"Honey," thought Charlie, "very nice. Probably lives in a big house with a rich husband. Ain't got to work, so spends her spare time sending idiots like me to prison. Wouldn't mind being banged up with her for a few months."

The prosecution opened proceedings. The solicitor wanted justice to be served. Society has had enough of people behaving in a manner which affects other members of the community.

"So you see," concluded the prosecution, "although these offences of dishonesty are not at the most serious end of the scale, they demonstrate a complete disregard for law and order."

Mr. Gordon stood up and cleared his throat.

"I would like to submit a psychiatrist's report to the bench. Dr. King has been treating my client for a number of years, and I feel his assessment is invaluable."

Mr. Gordon handed three copies of the report to the usher. They were passed to the bench. Silence fell.

"Lard-boy doesn't appear to be concentrating," thought Charlie, watching the man in the middle, "probably hoping he's got chips for tea."

Charlie glanced at Honey, who was reading intently.

"Wonder if she puts as much effort into her bedroom performance," he mused, "I'd love to find out."

Pin-head stopped reading and looked at Mr. Gordon.

"As you can see," said Mr. Gordon, "my client is in much greater need of help than punishment. With the correct help, I really believe that he could stop this pattern of offending."

"Thank-you," said Lard-boy, "we shall retire to consider sentence."

Charlie waited, fidgeting with the clips on his dungarees. Twenty minutes passed. He still waited.

"Fuck this," he thought, "how difficult can it be?"

Forty minutes passed. Charlie still waited.

"I don't believe this," he thought, "Lard-boy and Pin-head must be getting frisky with my Honey."

The bell rang. It had taken nearly an hour.

"Mr. Lloyd, please stand," ordered Lard-boy.

Charlie stood up, staring to his front.

"We have listened very carefully to your defence and studied intently Dr. King's detailed report. We have decided that help and guidance are the most appropriate way to prevent further offending. Do you agree to a probation order for two years?"

"Yes," answered Charlie.

"In addition," continued Lard-boy, "you shall be required to attend appointments with Dr. King as a condition of your probation."

"I will," said Charlie, "thank-you."

A CRY FOR EVER

"You are free to leave," concluded Lard-boy.

Charlie, walking on air, joined his mother at the back of the courtroom.

"Brilliant," he thought. "Now, all I've got to worry about is looking after Charlotte."

They left the court buildings.

"Last time I'm coming here," said Charlie.

"I do hope so," answered Hazel. "Come on, it'll only take a few minutes to get to the car park."

They hurried down the street. Two policeman, one short and fat, the other tall and thin, brushed passed them.

"Little and Large," thought Charlie. "Not going to have anything else to do with them."

They crossed the road, narrowly avoiding a speeding lorry. Then they walked through a garage forecourt, turned the corner and nearly collided with two lady pensioners.

"Did I hit the lady with the shopping bags?"

Charlie turned and watched as the two ladies headed for the town.

"They're fine," he reasoned, "they didn't give you a second look."

"Hurry up," said Hazel, "what's the matter?"

"Nothing," replied Charlie, staring at the pensioners.

"Come on, then," said Hazel.

"Okay," answered Charlie, watching the ladies until the last possible moment.

He turned and walked with Hazel. Charlie, anxious and agitated, didn't speak to his mother. He, for the moment, lived in his own world. A private, lonely and depressing place.

"It's okay," thought Charlie, "you watched them for as long as possible. You don't need to worry. They were fine."

They reached the car park and found Hazel's car.

"Come on," thought Charlie, "you have to stop doubting yourself. You didn't do anything wrong. Just try and focus on Charlotte. You've got more important things in your life than worrying about something that didn't happen."

Hazel drove Charlie to Linda's house.

"Got to stop worrying," decided Charlie, tapping on the door, "must concentrate on what's important....... Tiger."

Chapter 5

The weeks flew by. One Monday, the British weather, as it often did, kept Charlie and Charlotte indoors. They coloured while watching 'Noddy' on video.

"This is really good," mused Charlie, watching Charlotte scribble across the page. "I feel useful. At last I'm doing something worthwhile, something important. I've got a massive reason to fight the intrusive thoughts and resist any temptation to go back to prison."

It was early evening, and the rain pelted down even harder. Lucy, home from work, was reading Charlotte a bedtime story.

"The end," said Lucy, shutting the book.

"I'll take her to bed," said Charlie, "she looks really tired."

Charlie lay Charlotte gently, in her cot, kissed her cheek and sat in the doorway of the bedroom.

"Goodnight, Tiger," he whispered, "sweet dreams."

It wasn't long, a matter of minutes, before soft, regular breathing suggested Charlotte's day had come to an end.

Charlie, quietly, stood up and crept into the kitchen.

Lucy sat at the table, reading and drinking a cup of coffee.

"Tiger's asleep," said Charlie. "What are you reading?"

"Oh, a customer left this magazine at work," replied Lucy, "do you want to have a look at it?"

Charlie flicked through the glossy pages.

"I lost six stones in a year," he read. "My boyfriend slept with my mother." "My girlfriend left me for another woman."

He turned page after page.

"My husband infected me with HIV."

"I've spent seventy thousand pounds on plastic surgery."

He carried on browsing.

"I was terrified for my daughter..... but it was me with cancer!"

"Bloody hell," thought Charlie, "wonder what that's about."

He read the article.

"A single mother, who was struggling to look after her daughter, was diagnosed with bowel cancer . The father had left when she was pregnant and she had no relatives in a position to help. She was terrified the child would be put into care."

"That's awful," thought Charlie, "really awful."

"Wouldn't it be terrible if I got ill," he thought, "Then I wouldn't be able to look after Charlotte."

"Hang on," he panicked, "I'm not going to start thinking like that."

He went to make a coffee.

"You okay?" Lucy asked.

"Yeah," answered Charlie, "why do you ask?"

"You look a bit pale," answered Lucy, "that's all."

"What if I've got a serious illness?" Charlie thought.

"I just can't shift these bloody thoughts," he panicked, "I mustn't let someone else being ill affect me so badly."

The days, with Charlotte, were good. The weather, with wind and rain, wasn't. One afternoon, Charlie washed up the dinner plates as Charlotte tried, unsuccessfully, to build a tower from blocks.

"Don't worry, Tiger," he said, as the blocks collapsed, "try again."

A car stopped outside the house.

"Probably Lucy," thought Charlie, looking at the clock, "just finished work."

"Hi," said Lucy, chirpily, "how's Lottie today?"

"She's fine," answered Charlie, "well behaved, as always."

Lucy sat at the table.

"How was work?" Charlie asked.

"Hardly done any work today," answered Lucy. "I've been talking to Sharon, our accountant."

"Oh?" Charlie said.

"Well," continued Lucy, "Sharon has a friend, Mandy. Known her since primary school. Anyway, Mandy has a son; think he's about three or four."

"Yeah?" Charlie said.

"This lad, Alfie, ate some dog-muck," continued Lucy.

"Eh?" Charlie said.

"I'm not exactly sure what happened," continued Lucy, "he must have got the muck on his hands and put his hands in his mouth."

"And?" Charlie said.

"The little lad went blind," said Lucy.

"Are you sure?" Charlie asked.

"Yes," answered Lucy, "it's a condition called toxo……… um ……… something or other."

"That's so terrible," said Charlie, "how sad."
Charlie had never met Alfie, or even Mandy, so his trembling; shallow, rapid breathing; eyes failing to focus; racing heart rate and general agitation might have seemed a slight over-reaction.

That evening, as the wind howled in the trees outside the house, Charlie sat with Charlotte as she fought the urge to sleep.
"That poor kid," pondered Charlie, for the hundredth time, "I just can't believe it."
It wasn't long before Charlotte's soft, regular breathing signalled her defeat.
"What a life," thought Charlie, "all she has to worry about is her next meal, a clean nappy and a warm place to sleep."
He walked out of the bedroom and went straight to the bookshelf at the end of the hall. The medical dictionary sat on the bottom shelf next to 'A History of Effingham'.
"Shouldn't think this has been read for ages," he thought, taking the medical book.
It wasn't long before he found it – "Toxocariasis".
He read with intense interest, equalled by intense anxiety.
"A thread-like worm that lives in the intestines of dogs that can infest humans."
Charlie studied the rest of the information on the illness.
"So it could be true," he panicked, "the little boy could have gone blind if the worm was in the dog's muck."
He put the medical book on the shelf, hand a little unsteady. His head throbbed, adding to his agitation.
He recalled watching the evening news, many years earlier,.
"The battered old lady," he thought, "I remember the picture as if I'd seen it today. That was the beginning of the end of my 'normal' living. It would be so easy to compare my life then and now."

He plodded into the kitchen. If there's a problem......... drink a coffee and smoke a roll-up.
"Get a grip," he thought, "for fuck's sake."
He took a sip of the hot coffee.
"But," he panicked, "what if I went blind? I'd be no use to Charlotte. What if she went blind? It'd be my fault. Oh, fuck..... fuck......."
He took a drag on his roll-up.

"Calm down," he panicked, "it's very rare. The medical book said it wasn't a common problem."

Charlie gulped his coffee, scalding his throat.

"But it could happen," he worried, "I'm going to have to be so careful."

It was Wednesday morning, bright and chilly. Charlotte, after much persuasion, had finished a healthy breakfast.

"Come on, Tiger," said Charlie, "we've got to go to the shop to get some ham and beans."

Charlie strapped Charlotte in her pushchair.

"It should only take us about ten minutes to walk to the shops," he said.

He pushed Charlotte along the road.

"At least it's not raining," he thought.

They passed two horses grazing in a field.

"They look fed up," said Charlie, "still, they do spend all day in the same place."

Charlotte looked around, surveying her surroundings. Charlie walked purposefully, eyes to the front.

What's that?" Charlie wondered, noticing something on the pavement, about fifteen yards ahead.

He walked on, eyes fixed on the same spot. He must have been about nine or ten yards away.

"Oh no," he panicked, "it's bloody dog's muck."

He came to an abrupt halt. Rooted to the pavement, hands on the pushchair.

"You could go blind. You could cause Charlotte to go blind."

He stayed still, gripping the pushchair.

"Keep calm," he urged, "you ain't anywhere near the shit."

Charlie, dragging the pushchair, took a couple of backward paces. Then, he turned and walked back towards home.

"We won't be having ham and beans for lunch, "said Charlie to Charlotte, "we'll have to see what's in the cupboard."

Charlie, anxious and agitated, tried to regain some sort of control.

"My heart's going wild," he panicked, "my legs feel like jelly. Bloody hell, hope I don't collapse."

He walked slowly, concentrating on each movement. As he distanced himself from the offending dog's mess, his anxiety levels began to drop.

Back home, he relaxed considerably, although he felt angry

and disappointed.

"I'm sorry we didn't get to the shop, Tiger," said Charlie, "I feel awful about it."

Charlotte had a drink of blackcurrant and Charlie, as usual, a cup of hot coffee. He sat at the table while Charlotte played on the kitchen floor, oblivious to any problem.

"Why can't people clear up after their dogs," pondered Charlie, "how difficult would it be?"

He rolled a cigarette. Coffee without a smoke……. imagine that!

"Sure you didn't touch the poo?"

Charlie shook his head.

"I really don't need this," he panicked, "what is it trying to do to me?"

"What if you trod in the poo? Then you could have got it on your hands. What if you touched Charlotte and got some poo on her?"

Charlie sat still, not even bothering to smoke or drink.

"Don't let this thing destroy you," he urged, "you were at least ten yards away from the dog mess. There is no way you could have got any on you. No way."

Minutes ticked by and anxiety lowered. A throbbing pain across Charlie's forehead reminded him of the encounter.

Charlotte prodding Charlie's face told him another day had begun.

"Coffee," he murmured, heading for the kitchen.

He sat at the table as Charlotte munched her toast. He reflected on the previous day.

"That dog's mess caused me as much anxiety as an old woman," he mused, "but I mustn't give up. I can't just stay at home in case I come across some dog's muck. If I let it beat me…….. what about Charlotte?"

He looked at Charlotte. She'd finished her toast and marmite. Now she tackled a strawberry yogurt.

"Okay, Tiger," said Charlie, "when you're ready we're going to the shop. Hope you fancy ham and beans."

He pushed Charlotte along the road. The two horses still grazed in the field.

"What a boring life," thought Charlie again.

Then he, with rising anxiety, approached yesterday's spot.

"Keep calm," he urged, "if the dog's muck is still there, just walk in the road."

He walked on……. cautiously.

"No sign of it," he noted, "not a trace. Brilliant."

He walked on…….. anxiety lowering.

"Come on, Tiger," said Charlie, "we're nearly there."

Charlie pushed Charlotte into the shop. There was plenty of space for a pushchair.

"They sell everything in here," he thought, looking round the shop, "you can get anything you want."

Charlie picked up some sliced ham, a couple of tins of baked beans and a carton of orange juice. He joined the short queue behind a casually dressed, middle-aged lady.

"She won't be long," thought Charlie, looking in her basket, "only got a couple of cans of dog food."

He smiled at Charlotte sitting in the pushchair.

"Dog food. Must have a dog. Could have dog's mess on her."

Charlie, heart hammering, struggled for reality.

"Don't be so stupid," he panicked, "you're going mad."

Charlie, reluctantly, replaced his goods and, hurriedly, pushed Charlotte out the shop.

"Come on, Tiger," he said, "we'll come back later."

He headed for home.

"What the fuck was that all about?" he panicked, "you're losing the plot."

A few minutes from home, and his anxiety levels weren't much above normal.

But he couldn't help thinking, "The lady in the shop. Did you brush against her coat? Is it possible a toxocariasis worm got on you?"

He arrived home, trying to keep a grip on his anxiety. He headed straight for the bathroom.

"Hang on, Tiger," he said, "won't be long."

He scrubbed his hands, again and again. As the soap and water cleansed his skin, Charlie's anxiety lowered. Five minutes of washing and he started to relax.

He left the bathroom, a cleansed man. Free from the threat of blindness.

Days later, and Charlie stood at the bathroom sink washing his hands….. again. A few minutes earlier he had touched a stone in the garden.

"What if there was dog's muck on the stone?"

He held his hands under the taps, rinsing the last of the soap.

"This is bollocks," he thought, "I'm washing my hands about a hundred times every day. Every time I touch something that hasn't been sterilised, I have to go and wash my hands in case I go blind."

"Sorry, Tiger," said Charlie, back in the kitchen, "my hands were a bit grubby. Do you want to watch a video?"

The following day dawned clear and bright.

"Not a cloud in sight," said Charlie, putting Charlotte's breakfast plate in the sink, "let's go to the park."

Charlie made Charlotte a drink, strapped her in the pushchair, then took his knife from the top of the wardrobe.

"Always carry a knife," he thought, pocketing the folded weapon, "ever since I was attacked."

They spent a lovely morning playing on the swings.

"Better get home, Tiger," said Charlie, "you'll be wanting some lunch."

After eating, Charlie and Charlotte watched cartoons on the television. A knock on the door interrupted the programme.

"Hello," said Richard, "got a free day from college so thought I'd come and see you."

"Come in," said Charlie, "do you want a coffee?"

Charlie and Richard downed their third cup of coffee. Charlotte was quiet; cartoons seemed to have that effect.

"Richard lives in a house with two dogs. What if you touched his hand when you handed him his cup?"

Charlie tried to hide his agitation. This proved very difficult.

"You okay?" Richard asked.

"Fine," answered Charlie, "just need a piss."

Charlie stood up quickly and went to the bathroom. He washed his hands. It was almost ten minutes before his anxiety returned to a manageable level. He returned to the kitchen.

"You took your time," said Richard.

"I know," answered Charlie, "reckon I'm a bit constipated."

"Shall we have another cup?" Richard suggested.

"Er…. okay" answered Charlie.

He took two clean cups from the cupboard and made the drinks.

"I don't mind the same cup," said Richard.

"Don't worry," replied Charlie, "I enjoy washing up."

Charlie put Richard's drink on the table.

"No contact," thought Charlie, "nothing to worry about."

"Can I nick a roll-up off you?" Richard asked, sipping his drink.

"Er.......... yeah.......sure," replied Charlie, putting his tobacco in front of Richard.

There was the faintest brush of hands as Richard took the tobacco.

"Bollocks," thought Charlie, "what shit luck."

Richard lit his roll-up and inhaled deeply.

Charlie struggled to keep his composure. He kept his hands as far from his mouth as possible.

"Mustn't put my hands near my face," he panicked, "if I've got one of those bastard worms on me, don't want to get it in my mouth."

Charlie gripped his hands together, stretched, away from him, across the table. He must have looked quite strange.

"You okay, mate?" Richard asked, for the second time.

"Shoulders aching," replied Charlie, keeping his arms tense and to the front.

"Oh," said Richard.

"Surely, I don't need to wash again," thought Charlie.

As he sat at the table, arms outstretched, he became more and more agitated and anxious.

"Crap," thought Charlie, "if I don't wash my hands...... I won't be able to concentrate on fuck-all else."

He stood up, arms still stretched away from his body.

"Need the toilet, again," he said to Richard, "don't know what the fuck is wrong with me."

He hurried, almost running, to the bathroom. As the soap and water went to work, his anxiety fell away.

Charlie sat opposite Dr. King. Another Wednesday, another appointment at the clinic.

"So," said Dr. King, "how did you get here, today?"

"My mum gave me a lift," answered Charlie, "she's in the waiting room with Charlotte."

"So, how are things?" Dr. King asked.

"Well," replied Charlie, "I've been very worried about an illness - toxocariasis. I heard these worms, found in dog's muck, could make you go blind."

"And?" Dr. King asked.

"Whenever I go near dog's muck or a dog or, even, somebody who owns a dog, I feel terrible," answered Charlie.

"Can you explain?" asked the doctor.

"I feel really stressed, "said Charlie, "I get really agitated. I can't concentrate on anything else."

"So, what do you do?" Dr. King asked.

"I have to wash my hands," replied Charlie, "I've been washing my hands all the time."

"And this helps?" Dr. King asked.

"Yeah," replied Charlie, "when I've washed my hands I feel normal again."

"Are you still taking your medication?" the doctor asked.

"Yeah," answered Charlie.

"Is it helping?"

"I think so," replied Charlie, "the pills take the edge off the worries."

"So, what if you don't wash your hands?"

"I can't cope," answered Charlie.

"Okay," said Dr. King, "there's no quick fix but, for now, I would like you to resist the urge to wash for as long as possible. With time, this will show you that failing to wash your hands will not result in your going blind."

"I'll try," said Charlie, doubtfully.

"And keep taking the same dose," added the doctor.

"Right," said Charlie, "will do."

"See you next week," concluded Dr. King.

Saturday morning was overcast but dry. Charlie, with Charlotte strapped in the pushchair, walked to Linda's house. Charlotte always seemed really pleased to see her mother.

"See you Monday, Tiger," he said, waving from the gate, "have a lovely time."

The following day, mid-afternoon, Charlie lay on his bed listening to the radio. The phone rung in the next room.

"Better answer it," he decided, "might be important."

"Hello, mate," said Edward, instantly recognisable.

"Hello," said Charlie, "how's life with you?"

"Okay," answered Edward, "same as ever."

"Good," said Charlie.

"There's something I thought you should know," said

Edward.

"Yeah?"

"Last night," said Edward, "I was on my way home from The Windsor. Totally pissed. Anyway, I walked past Linda's place just before midnight."

"Yeah?"

"Clive Chew," continued Edward, "and three or four of his mates were going into the house."

"Oh," said Charlie.

"Was Charlotte staying at Linda's last night?"

"Yeah," answered Charlie.

"Well," continued Edward, "they were carrying tins and, from what I could tell, were already totally lashed."

"Right," said Charlie.

"I wouldn't have it," said Edward, "if my daughter was there, I wouldn't want that lot drinking all night."

"Yeah, I see," said Charlie.

"I'd have a word with him," said Edward, "I think it's totally out of order."

"Maybe I should," replied Charlie.

"If you want me to come with you," said Edward, "or phone him……"

"Let me have a think," answered Charlie.

"Okay," said Edward, "speak to you later."

Charlie sat at the kitchen table, roll-up in one hand and coffee in the other.

"It ain't good," he pondered, "spliced blokes going round Linda's after the pub when Charlotte is there. Reckon Ed's got a point - have to say something."

He dragged on the skinny roll-up.

"Clive Chew," he thought, "I remember him. Tall, dark hair, hooked nose and staring eyes. Not desperately attractive. Think he works in the building trade. Lives near The Anchor."

Charlie sipped his coffee.

"Right," he decided, "I'll have a word."

He picked up the phone and dialed Ed's number.

"Hello, Ed," said Charlie, "can you come round?"

"Okay," replied Edward, "be there in a bit."

Edward and Charlie sat at the table, drinking and smoking.

"We'll have a chat with Clive," said Charlie, "just to let him know the score."

"I reckon we should," replied Edward.

"Nothing serious," said Charlie, "just to warn him."

"Okay," said Edward.

"We could even phone him," said Charlie, "ain't got to be done face to face."

"No time like the present, "said Edward, "I'll call him now."

They found his phone number in the directory. Twenty rings but no answer.

"Lives on his own," said Edward, replacing the receiver, "we might as well walk round his house."

"Well......." answered Charlie, "if he's there, we could talk to him. Just talk, nothing else."

"Come on, then," said Edward.

Charlie took his knife from the wardrobe.

"Won't need this," he thought, "but I never leave home without it."

They pressed the bell and waited.

"Might not be working," said Edward, knocking on the door.

No answer. Clive wasn't home or didn't want visitors.

"Bollocks," cursed Edward, "we'll try again soon."

Monday, mid-morning, and Charlotte was home.

"What do you want to do," Charlie asked, "read a book or watch a video?"

He turned another page of the book he was reading, and read on.

The phone rang, interrupting the story.

"Hello," said Edward, "I'm not doing much today. Do you fancy popping round?"

"I've got Charlotte," answered Charlie.

"That's fine," said Edward, "bring her with you."

"Okay," replied Charlie, "we'll be round in a while."

He strapped Charlotte in the pushchair, made her a drink, put the knife in his pocket and left the house.

They didn't hurry; it wasn't far and Edward wasn't going anywhere.

"Three horses in the field, Tiger," he said , "an extra one."

They crossed the road and passed the school, then walked up a slope and turned the corner.

"Hello, Charlie."

Charlie looked at the two men standing in front of him.

"Fuck me," he thought, "Clive Chew and his mate, James

A CRY FOR EVER

Wiseman."

James Wiseman lived locally. Short and stocky, he was proud of his muscular build, which would explain his preference for sleeveless tops, even in the cold.

"If I don't say anything," he thought, "I probably never will. Not to mention looking a right cock."

He put Charlotte, in her pushchair, back round the corner.

"Hope nothing kicks off," thought Charlie, "I didn't expect Clive to have a mate with him."

He walked towards the two men, taking out his knife and opening the blade.

"Want a word with you," he said, looking at Clive.

"What about?" Clive answered.

"Linda's ain't a drop-in centre," snarled Charlie, "you can't go round there if you fancy a drink. Charlotte was upstairs."

"What are you going to do," said Clive, "stab me?"

"Is he taking the piss?" Charlie thought.

He held the blade at Clive's neck. Not enough pressure to cut the skin, just enough to leave a mark.

"Shit," thought Charlie, "have I cut him or stabbed him - fuck knows."

Charlie shot a glance at Wiseman. He hadn't moved; he just observed the scene.

"If I stab him," thought Charlie, "anything could happen. Wiseman could get involved. He ain't gonna stand there and watch his mate get knifed."

"Okay," said Clive, "I ain't bothered about going round there."

"Thank fuck for that," thought Charlie, "sorted."

He slowly pulled away the knife from Clive's neck. He walked round the corner folding the blade, then slipped it into his pocket. He grabbed the pushchair and walked..... quickly.

Cars passed in both directions.

"Blimey," pondered Charlie, "at least ten drivers would have seen what happened. I just want to get to Edward's house...... quickly."

He hurried along, almost running.

"Hope Clive leaves it at that," he thought, "could do without any more hassle."

It was only a matter of minutes before Charlie knocked on Edward's door.

"Guess who I've just seen," said Charlie, standing on the

doorstep, "Clive and one of his mates. Had a word with Clive..... pulled a blade on him."

"Didn't use it?" Edward asked.

"No," replied Charlie.

"Shit," said Edward, staring down the road.

"What's the matter?" Charlie asked, turning round.

A police car had parked a few houses along the street.

"Fuck, fuck," cursed Charlie.

"Don't panic," said Edward, "just give me the knife."

"I can't get it out," said Charlie "it's too obvious."

"Come in the house," said Edward.

Charlie took Charlotte from the pushchair. Two policeman got out of their car and, without giving Charlie and Edward a second glance, walked into a neighbouring property.

"Panic over," said Edward, "they've gone to see Chris Gould. He's always in trouble."

"Thank fuck," said Charlie, stumbling into Ed's kitchen, "put the kettle on. I need a coffee."

A few hours later, arriving back home, Charlie flopped at the kitchen table. Charlotte, perfectly contented, emptied the cupboards onto the floor.

"My calf muscle feels a bit odd," thought Charlie, rubbing his leg, "a little bit of an ache."

He rolled a cigarette.

"I wonder what's wrong with my leg," he pondered, "probably nothing. Have just walked the best part of a couple of miles."

He dragged on the roll-up.

"It could be something really serious. What would you know? Could be a blood clot or something."

Charlie, trying not to panic, found reality a difficult concept.

"Don't be so bloody daft," he urged, "it's unlikely to be terminal."

He finished his roll-up, trying desperately, but failing miserably, to concentrate on anything but his aching calf.

"Okay, Tiger," he said, "here's your colouring book. Let's see how long it takes you to finish a picture."

He took the colouring book from the drawer and handed it to Charlotte. She had plenty of pens scattered around the floor.

"While you are doing that," he said, "I've got some reading to do."

He brought the medical dictionary to the kitchen table. Charlie scanned the pages with an unhealthy interest.

"Legs......." he murmured, "anything that could cause a pain in the leg."

He read about many conditions, illnesses and diseases.

"Bloody hell," he thought, "there is so much that can go wrong. I've never heard of most of these."

He turned another page.

"Buerger's disease," he read, "a disorder in which the arteries, nerves and veins become severely inflamed, causing pain in the legs and feet."

"Shit," he panicked, reading on.

"In severe cases, gangrene can result."

"Oh, fuck me,"he thought, trying to focus on the text, "fuck me."

"This condition mainly affects young men who smoke."

"Bollocks," he moaned.

He stopped reading; too much information for one day.

"Doubt I've got that," mused Charlie, "much more likely to be a pulled muscle."

He looked at Charlotte, happily colouring a blue tree.

"You've probably got Buerger's disease. You're young, male and a heavy smoker. You'll probably have both legs cut off. Won't be much use to Charlotte, will you?"

"No need to panic. I'll just see what happens."

Tuesday lunchtime on a fine, sunny day.

"What a nice morning, Tiger," said Charlie, taking her from the pushchair, "it's so much better when the weather is good and we can go to the swings."

He made Charlotte a drink and flicked on the kettle.

"Oh no," he thought, "my bloody calf is aching again."

He handed Charlotte her drink, desperately trying to hide his agitation. He slumped at the table, fighting to stay in control.

"This is no bloody good," he decided, "a pain in my leg is dominating my whole life."

He got the phone, checked the number and dialled.

"Hello, surgery."

"I'd like an appointment," said Charlie, "as soon as possible."

"How about tomorrow at twelve?"

"That's great," he answered, making a mental note to cancel his psychiatric appointment, "thank-you."

Wednesday, exactly twelve o'clock, and he was already in

the doctor's consulting room.

"I always thought doctors were late," he pondered.

Charlotte sat, in her pushchair, near the couch.

"What can I do for you?" Dr. Peacock asked.

He was a short man of slight build, aged around forty, with a brisk, no-nonsense approach.

"My leg hurts," stammered Charlie, "I often get a pain in my calf. I'm so worried about Buerger's disease."

"Take off your shoes and socks, please," said Dr. Peacock.

He felt Charlie's feet, taking a matter of seconds.

Charlie fought to stay in control. His whole life hung by a thread.

"You have a strong pulse in both feet, so there is no blockage," said Dr. Peacock, "certainly not Buerger's disease."

"You're absolutely sure?" Charlie asked.

"Yes," answered Dr. Peacock, "feel for yourself."

Charlie put a finger on his foot and the doctor guided it to the exact spot. He could feel his pulse, throbbing under his tentative finger. Other foot, same result.

"Thank-you," he said, "thank-you, so much."

Charlie felt an overwhelming desire to hug Dr. Peacock, such was his relief.

"Thank fuck," he thought, "what a wonderful man. Given me back my life. Saved me from losing my legs. Made sure I can look after Tiger."

Charlie, with pushchair, left the surgery.

"Feel like I've got a last minute reprieve from a death sentence," he thought, heading home, "now I can start living."

Chapter 6

Charlotte lived happily, day by day. Charlie fought his intrusions, hour upon hour. It was a Tuesday, and Charlotte's many toys were scattered across the kitchen floor.

"Come on, Tiger," he said, "let's go to the sweet shop. I'd like to get a newspaper and I reckon you'd like some sweets."

They walked past the park.

"Fancy a quick push on the swings?" he asked.

It was over an hour before they reached the newsagents'.

"Choose some sweets, Tiger," he said, "I'm just going to get

a paper and some tobacco."
Charlie paid the assistant and they left the shop. They walked past the park, across the road and turned into the home strait.
"Nearly there, Tiger," said Charlie, "only five more minutes."

A figure walked towards them, approaching from the other end of the road.
"Oh," thought Charlie, slightly uneasy, "an old woman."
He walked on, hands on the pushchair.
"This won't be a problem, Tiger," he said, "we'll be fine."
As they passed the lady, Charlie increased his grip on the pushchair and allowed her as much space as was possible.
"Good morning," he said, with a smile.
"Morning, dear," she replied.
A few yards further on, Charlie shot a quick glance behind him.
"She's fine," he thought, "and I didn't even worry. Only felt slightly anxious."

They reached home and Charlie unlocked the door.
"Postman' s been," he said, picking a letter from the floor, "looks important."
He opened the envelope.
"You've been given an appointment for a hearing test, Tiger," he said, "at Epsom Hospital. That was quick; the GP only referred you a couple of weeks ago."
Charlotte sat on the floor, sweets in one hand and puzzle in the other.

Meanwhile, Charlie sat at the table and opened his newspaper.
"Superbug in hospitals," screamed the headlines.
"Bloody hell," he panicked, reading the article, "what's this all about?"
"A flesh-eating bug," he read, "that enters the body through an open wound in the skin. This flesh-eating bug would, quickly, devour its host if doctors were unable to rid the body of the parasite. It is found, predominantly, in hospitals."
Charlie paced the kitchen floor, trying to be rational.
"Shit," he panicked, "what if you had an operation. This bug enters the body through open wounds. You're not going to get a bigger opening than that."

Charlie continued pacing, still trying to be rational.

"Oh no," he panicked, "what if I need my appendix taken out or something like that."

He slumped at the kitchen table.

"Oh no," he panicked for the second time in a minute, "I've got to go to Epsom Hospital next week. Tiger has got her hearing test."

Day followed night, and worry followed intrusion. A day before the hearing test, Charlie sat at the kitchen table, chain smoking and downing coffee after coffee. Charlotte played happily on the floor, unaware of his distress.

"Suppose I could cancel the appointment," he mused, "that'd solve the problem."

He rolled another cigarette.

"Can't do that," he decided, "what if there is a problem with Tiger's hearing. And, they'd only arrange it for another day."

That night, Charlotte slept peacefully, while Charlie sat in the kitchen. Lucy and Hazel had gone out.

"Must make sure that I haven't got any open wounds," thought Charlie, "don't want that fucking bug finding a way in."

He looked at both hands, front and back.

"Shit," he cursed, "I've got loads of tiny cuts. I'll have to cover every one. Can't take any chances."

He went to the medicine cabinet and, to his great relief, found a packet of plasters.

"Right," he decided, "in the morning, before I go to hospital, I'll put a plaster on every cut."

He opted for an early night, not wanting to oversleep the next day.

It was a bright, sunny morning. Charlie jumped out of bed, remembering he had a busy start to the day. Hazel and Charlotte were already sitting at the kitchen table, eating breakfast. Charlie smoked a roll-up and downed a cup of coffee. He went to the bathroom, washed his face and cleaned his teeth.

"Won't have a shave," he decided, "I don't want to risk cutting my face."

Charlie opened the medicine cabinet and took the plasters.

"Got a few cuts on my hands," he said to Hazel.

"Hurry up," answered Hazel, "I'm driving you to the hospital, we've got to leave soon."

"Okay," said Charlie, heading for his bedroom.

He sat on the bed.

"I'll cover every cut, however small," he thought "don't want to take any chances."

He stuck a couple of plasters on his fingers. He looked closely at his hands: a few cuts on his palms and several on the back of his hands. As he tried to cover a small cut on his palm, another plaster came unstuck.

"Shit," he cursed, "this ain't going to be easy."

He tried again, with little success. As fast as he stuck the plasters, others came loose.

"This is impossible," he thought, "there's no way I'll be able to cover every cut with plasters."

He paced the bedroom.

"I know," he thought, "gloves."

He rushed around the house looking for a pair of gloves.

"Must have some," he thought, searching a drawer in the kitchen.

"What are you doing?" Hazel asked.

"Oh, nothing," answered Charlie.

"Well, come on," said Hazel, "or we are going to be late."

"Okay," said Charlie, "just a second."

He had another look in his wardrobe. Nothing.

"Shit," he panicked, "what the hell am I going to do?"

He went back to the kitchen. Hazel and Charlotte were waiting by the door.

"Washing-up gloves," he thought, looking at the sink.

He grabbed the gloves.

"They're bright pink," he thought, "I'm going to look a right wanker. Still, got to cover the cuts on my hands."

"Why are you wearing those gloves?" Hazel asked, as they drove towards Epsom.

"Oh……. um ……….no reason," stammered Charlie.

"You look a bit of an idiot," said Hazel.

"Look," answered Charlie, "it's my choice."

Charlie, his mother and his daughter, went through the hospital to the ENT department.

Two ladies, middle-aged and smartly dressed, hurried along the corridor. They were laughing and joking - unusual behaviour in a hospital. All of a sudden, they fell silent. They were staring at Charlie's gloves, bright pink, washing-up gloves.

"Oh no," thought Charlie, "this is so embarrassing. But, it's got to be better than getting eaten alive."

He stared at the two women. They glanced at one another and walked on. Charlie could hear them talking and laughing after they had turned the corner at the end of the corridor.

"At least they've got something to laugh about, now," pondered Charlie.

"ENT," said Hazel, pointing at a sign, "we're here."

The waiting room was busy, so it was a great relief to be seen quickly. A couple of teenage girls found Charlie's appearance most comical. Charlotte's ENT doctor, Dr. Morris, glanced at Charlie only slightly longer than necessary.

"You okay?" he asked.

"Fine, thank-you," answered Charlie.

The appointment was short and sweet. Charlotte's hearing was perfect. Driving out of the hospital car park, Charlie removed the gloves.

"So glad that's over," he thought, "no worries."

One Thursday afternoon, as rain pelted down outside, Charlie and Charlotte were colouring at the kitchen table.

There was a sharp knock at the back door.

"Wonder who that could be," said Charlie, standing up.

"Hello," grinned Andrew, Lucy's boyfriend, "is Lucy in?"

"Still at work," answered Charlie.

"Can I wait for her?" asked Andrew, who was tall and thin with protruding ears and a gormless expression.

"Okay," answered Charlie.

He left the door open and walked back in to the kitchen.

"Surprised Lucy and Andrew have lasted the last two months," he pondered, "he might be an office manager, but what a tosser. Rather be in solitary confinement than with him."

Charlie, Andrew and Charlotte had been sitting at the table for nearly an hour. The conversation wasn't exactly flowing.

"Where's Lucy," thought Charlie, "I can't stand this pillock for much longer."

A CRY FOR EVER

"Can I have some cheese?" Charlotte asked.

"Yeah," replied Charlie, standing up, "I'll get you some."

He handed her a slice of cheese. She took a small bite, didn't like the flavour and spat it out.

"That's really naughty, Charlotte," snapped Andrew.

"Don't worry about it," said Charlie, "she obviously doesn't like it."

Lucy came home from work. She took Andrew into the lounge.

"Who the fuck does he think he is," thought Charlie, "speaking to Charlotte like that. Fucking stuck up cunt!"

Charlie and Charlotte carried on with their picture, but Charlie couldn't concentrate, his thoughts being elsewhere.

Charlie missed Charlotte every weekend.

"I'm always knackered when she's here," he thought, one Saturday afternoon, "but bored when she's with Linda."

He sat in the kitchen, puffing on a roll-up. Hazel and Lucy had gone shopping.

It was a few hours later when a car stopped outside the house. Lucy and Hazel struggled into the kitchen overloaded with shopping bags.

"Hello," said Lucy, "what have you been doing?"

"Nothing much," answered Charlie.

He rolled another cigarette.

"I was thinking," Charlie said to Lucy, "haven't seen Andrew for a while. What's happened to him?"

"Oh," answered Lucy, "he met some girl in a pub. Won't be seeing him again."

"You're not bothered?" Charlie asked.

"Best rid," answered Lucy.

Hazel and Lucy finished putting away their many purchases.

"Got to go out again," said Hazel, "going to visit Auntie Ivy."

"Okay," said Charlie, "see you later."

He stayed at the kitchen table, deciding whether to make a coffee.

"That fucking Andrew," thought Charlie, for the hundredth time that hour, "got to do something about him."

He paced the kitchen floor. After twenty or thirty lengths, an idea started to take shape.

He found a phone number written in his book, picked up the receiver and dialled. His mind wandered as he waited for

Anna to answer.

"I remember meeting her in the bus shelter on the way home from Ed's house, years ago," thought Charlie. "Tall girl, eighteen, red hair and freckles. Not a bad figure. Quite attractive, in fact. We got talking and realised we knew lots of the same people. She came back with me. A quick grope in the garden shed, interrupted by irreversible damage to Hazel's new lawnmower when I tripped over a rake."

Still no answer.

"Romance hasn't blossomed," pondered Charlie, "but we did stay in contact. Have gone months, even years, without speaking, but I always felt able to ring her."

"Hello," said Anna.

"Hi," said Charlie, "guess who."

They chatted for over an hour; there was plenty to talk about.

"I was after a favour," said Charlie, finally.

"Oh," replied Anna.

"I wanted a lift," said Charlie, "late at night."

"You're not stealing again?" Anna asked.

"No," answered Charlie, "it's not strictly legal, but I certainly wouldn't ask you to take stolen goods in your car."

"So, what is it?" Anna asked.

"Best if I don't say anything," answered Charlie, "but I'll make sure that you don't get into any trouble."

"I must be mad," said Anna, "but, okay."

"Thank-you," said Charlie, "very much."

Later that day, Charlie went to his local hardware store and made a single purchase. That evening, he sat in his bedroom and scribbled a few carefully- selected words on a piece of paper.

Saturday evening, a week later, Charlie and Anna sat in the lounge watching the television. Hazel and Lucy were both staying with a relative who hadn't been well. Around two o'clock in the morning, Charlie took his jacket from the peg, checked he had what was needed and went to the door. Anna followed, reluctantly.

"Where are we going?" Anna asked.

"Just stop here," answered Charlie, pointing at a space along the road.

He got out the car.

"Wait here," he said, "won't be long."

A CRY FOR EVER

He stood outside Andrew's house. Andrew's car was parked in the driveway, near the building.

"Let's do it," he murmured.

He took a tin of paint stripper from his pocket, pushed down on the lid and turned it. He crept towards Andrew's car, keeping an eye on the house.

"Don't want anyone looking out of the window," he thought.

He poured the stripper onto the back of the car, the roof, not forgetting the bonnet. He took a crumpled piece of paper from his pocket and placed it by the wheel. He put a small stone on the paper to stop it blowing away. He walked away from the house, empty tin of stripper in his hand.

"All done," said Charlie to Anna, opening the car door.

"What's that?" Anna asked, pointing at the tin.

"Let's get going," replied Charlie, "and I'll tell you."

When they had travelled a couple of miles, Charlie wiped the empty tin with a tissue and threw it out the window.

"So, what have you done?" Anna asked.

"Well," answered Charlie, "nothing serious as I don't want to go back to prison now I've got Charlotte. I paint-stripped Andrew's car."

"Oh," said Anna.

"And," added Charlie, "I left a note by the car."

"Why? What did it say?"

"Told Andrew I'd see him again, very soon," answered Charlie.

"Why did you put that?" Anna asked.

"I want him to worry," answered Charlie.

"He'll call the police," said Anna, "and give them the note."

"I don't reckon he will," replied Charlie, "he'll call the police so he can claim the insurance but I don't think he'll mention the note."

"Why?"

"Even though he's got a posh job," answered Charlie, "he's a bit of a dodgy fucker. He won't want the police involved. I reckon he'll come round and try and smooth things over."

"What will you do?" Anna asked.

"Have to wait and see," answered Charlie.

Life flew by, day after day. Hazel and Lucy had taken Charlotte to visit relatives. Charlie sat at the kitchen table, listening to the radio, drinking a cup of coffee.

"Boring without Tiger," he pondered, "might as well have a

kip. Just have one last fag."

He opened the tobacco.

"As soon as I've smoked this, I'll go to bed for a while."

There was a knock on the door.

"Wonder who that could be," thought Charlie.

He took a long drag, then put his roll-up in the ashtray.

"It's open," he shouted.

The door opened and Andrew walked into the room.

"Hello, mate," said Andrew.

Charlie didn't answer. He stood up and walked towards Andrew.

"Now or never," he thought, "this is what I've planned. Be a shame not to make the most of the opportunity."

Charlie paced across the kitchen.

"Suppose I could talk to him," he pondered. "He's got no proof about his car."

A few more steps.

"No," decided Charlie, "he's going to get it. Think of Charlotte."

Charlie aimed a right hook at Andrew's face. Andrew moved his head at exactly the perfect moment. The blow glanced across his face, having little effect. Andrew grabbed Charlie around his waist and clung on.

"Calm down," cried Andrew.

Charlie grabbed Andrew's head and forced it downwards. He forcibly lifted his knee; Andrew's face and head were the target area.

"Leave it," moaned Andrew, loosening his grip on Charlie.

Charlie lashed, repeatedly, at the side of Andrew's face.

"'Bout time," he thought.

Andrew sank to the floor, desperately trying to cover his head and face.

"Please....." he whispered.

Charlie grabbed Andrew, taking handfuls of designer clothing, and forced him out of the door. A final effort, and Andrew lay on the porch floor, one side of his face already swollen.

"Why......" Andrew moaned, blood oozing from his eye.

"Just leave," snarled Charlie, "fuck off and don't come back."

Charlie, quietly, closed the kitchen door and left Andrew, outstretched on the floor.

"Really hate things like that," thought Charlie, pacing the kitchen.

He sat at the table and rolled a cigarette. His hands were slightly unsteady.

"Can't fucking believe I'm shaking," he thought. "It was only Andrew. He ain't exactly a local heavyweight."

He heard footsteps outside the house.

"Must be Andrew going," he thought, "least he ain't too badly hurt."

It was a breezy Friday afternoon. Charlie and Charlotte sat in the doctor's waiting room…….. again.

"Shouldn't be long, Tiger," said Charlie, glancing at the clock.

Dr. Eastburn walked into the waiting area.He was a short man with thick glasses and grey hair.

"Not exactly a heart-throb," pondered Charlie. "Still, if he knows his stuff, who cares?"

"Charlie Lloyd, please," said Dr. Eastburn, "follow me."

Charlie, with Charlotte tagging behind, followed the doctor into his room.

"What can I do for you?" Dr. Eastburn asked.

"I'm really worried I've got gangrene," spluttered Charlie.

"Really?" Dr. Eastburn said, raising his eyebrows.

"I think so," said Charlie.

"Where?" Dr. Eastburn asked.

"On my arm," replied Charlie, showing a small, darkly-coloured mark.

"That's a bruise," said Dr. Eastburn. "It's definitely not gangrene."

"Are you sure?" Charlie asked.

"Certain," replied the doctor, "I'd stake my reputation on it."

"Thank fuck," thought Charlie, the knot loosening in his stomach. "He must think I'm such a cock. Still, I ain't going to have my arm amputated, so who gives a shit."

Charlie stood up. His anxiety level was normal, but he did feel slightly embarrassed.

"Thank-you so much," said Charlie, "I'm so grateful."

"That's okay," replied Dr. Eastburn, "but this is your third appointment this week and there hasn't been anything wrong with you. I would recommend talking about your fear of illnesses with your psychiatrist."

"I will, "said Charlie, taking Charlotte's hand and leading her to the door, "thanks again."

As it was a gloomy afternoon with the constant threat of rain, Charlie and Charlotte stayed indoors.

"Rather watch 'Winnie the Pooh' than get soaked at the park," thought Charlie.

A car pulled up outside the house.

"Must be nanny, home from work," said Charlie.

Charlie heard the back door open. Hazel walked into the lounge a few seconds later.

"Hello," said Hazel, "how about a coffee?"

"Lovely," answered Charlie.

Hazel prepared two cups of coffee, not forgetting a cold drink for Charlotte.

"Have you been to see the doctor lately?" Hazel asked.

"A few times," answered Charlie. "Think they're getting a bit pissed off with me."

"You're best bet would be to marry a doctor," said Hazel, "then you wouldn't have to keep running to the surgery."

"I wish," sighed Charlie.

"When is your next appointment with Dr. King?" Hazel asked.

"Few days," answered Charlie, "but I've got a probation appointment tomorrow."

"I'll be at work," said Hazel, "will you be able to get there?"

"Yeah," replied Charlie, "Anna said that she'll give me a lift."

"That's nice of her," said Hazel.

The following morning, Charlie and Charlotte had just finished breakfast when a car stopped outside the house.

Charlie headed for the door.

"Come on, Tiger," he said, "mustn't keep Mr. Carson waiting."

"Hello, Anna," said Charlie, opening the car door.

"Hi," said Anna. "I've brought Debbie with me. She wasn't working in the pub today, so she decided to come with us."

"Great," said Charlie.

Charlie and Charlotte climbed into the back of the car.

"Hello Debbie," said Charlie, "long time, no see."

"Been very busy," replied Debbie, "working at the pub and I've met a new chap."

"Oh," said Charlie, "who's that?"

"He's called Troy," replied Debbie, "lives in Guildford. He's very tall and, definitely, in proportion."

"Lovely," said Charlie, "has he got a job?"

"He does artwork for a magazine," replied Debbie, "earns loads of money."

"Blimey," thought Charlie, "Debbie has done well. Even though she's very petite, she does like tall men. And an artist....... quite a result. When I first met her, at Anna's house, she was knocking about with some overweight alcoholic."

The roads were quiet; they'd picked a good time to travel.

"Should be there in a few minutes," said Anna.

"We certainly ain't going to be late," said Charlie, scratching his shoulder.

Charlie pulled back his jumper so he could see what was itching.

"Been bitten, I expect," he thought.

He turned his head and peered at his left shoulder. A mole. Small, light brown. Definitely a mole.

"Could be a malignant melanoma!"

"Don't be so bloody stupid," thought Charlie, "it's a normal mole. Nothing more and nothing less."

"What if it's cancerous and it's spread!"

"Get a grip," panicked Charlie, staring at the offending mole.

"You could be riddled with cancer!"

"Think rationally," urged Charlie, fighting a desire to scream.

"Are you okay, Charlie?" Anna asked.

No reply. Charlie still sat in the back of the car but his mind was in hospital, having surgery, radiotherapy, final hours, funeral, Charlotte left alone.

"Are you okay?" Anna repeated.

"Um....... yeah," mumbled Charlie.

"Good," said Anna. "We're here."

Charlie sat opposite Mr. Carson, his probation officer. He was a stocky man, about six foot, trendy haircut and snappy dresser. Charlie heard what he was saying, but he wasn't really listening.

"So," said Mr. Carson, "I take it, you've been keeping out of trouble."

"What if I've got skin cancer," panicked Charlie, "I have read that a new mole can be a sign that something is wrong."

"So," said Mr. Carson, "how are things?"

"It's probably not even a new mole," pondered Charlie, "just haven't noticed it before."

Mr. Carson asked, "any developments?"

"What if you get a new mole and you don't notice? Could be cancer!"

"I got my secretary pregnant," said Mr. Carson, "do you reckon my wife will mind?"

"Sorry," said Charlie, trying to concentrate.

"Right," said Mr. Carson, "how's everything?"

"Not too bad," replied Charlie.

"Haven't been tempted to get into trouble?"

"No," answered Charlie.

"And you're still seeing Dr. King?"

"Yes," replied Charlie, "got an appointment in a couple of days."

"And Dr. King is still a great help?"

"Yes," replied Charlie.

"Okay," said Mr. Carson, "I'll see you again in a fortnight."

The journey home didn't last long, but seemed an eternity. Anna and Debbie chatted and laughed. Charlie stayed silent. Charlotte sat, chewing her sweets, looking out the window.

"Thanks for taking me," said Charlie, shutting the car door.

He went straight to the kitchen, found a pen, then headed to the bathroom.

"Won't be a minute, Tiger," he said, closing the door, "watch a video for a few minutes. Any problems, knock on the door."

He stood in front of the mirror and removed his jumper and dungarees.

"This is crazy," he thought, standing in a pair of shorts, "still, got to be done."

He circled every mole on his body. It was a struggle to reach certain places on his person.

"Don't think I've missed any on my back," he decided, straining to check.

He stared in the mirror, trying every possible angle.

"Now I can check to see if I have any new moles," he thought, "if I have a mole without a circle, I'll panic."

He dressed as quickly as possible.

"I can check as often as I want," he pondered, "and early detection is so important."

Charlie walked into the lounge. Jungle Book played on the television. Charlotte sat and watched, completely unaffected by any threat, real or unreal, from skin cancer.

It was raining heavily the following day.

A CRY FOR EVER

"Won't be able to go to the park, Tiger," said Charlie.

They chose a selection of puzzles.

"At least I can check for new moles," he thought, "I could hardly do that if I was at the park."

Two puzzles were completed on the kitchen floor.

"What if you got a new, cancerous mole!"

"Must check my body," he panicked.

He put a piece of puzzle on the floor.

"Won't be a minute, Tiger," he said, "carry on with the puzzle."

Charlie hurried to the bathroom, closed the door, stripped to his shorts, then checked his body.

"Looks okay," he pondered, "I'll do one final check."

The day passed quickly. Charlotte was good company and an invaluable distraction. But, when she was sleeping, he did a final check.

"Everything fine," he thought, "no worries."

He had a quick wash, then cleaned his teeth. It was on his final rinse that he noticed blood in the water. His gums were bleeding!

Charlie sat opposite Dr. King, relaxed by the psychiatrist's soothing tone.

"So," said Dr. King, "how are things?"

"I'm always worried that I've got some terrible illness," replied Charlie.

"What puts these ideas into your head?" Dr. King asked.

"Well," replied Charlie, "if I hear about a condition, I worry that it'll affect me and I won't be able to look after Charlotte."

"Is it one illness in particular?" Dr. King asked.

"No," replied Charlie, "I've been worried about loads of different complaints."

"Does this problem have an affect on your daily life?" Dr. King asked.

"Yes," replied Charlie. "I spend most of the day worrying that there is something wrong with me. I mean, one Tuesday, I spent several hours checking the pulse in my foot. I'm always reading the medical book trying to convince myself that I'm okay."

"Is anything bothering you at present?" Dr. King asked.

"Leukaemia," replied Charlie.

"Okay," said Dr. King, "why do you think you've got that?"

"Well," said Charlie, "I was brushing my teeth the other night and my gums started to bleed."

"Oh," said the doctor.

"Well," continued Charlie, "I looked in the medical book and bleeding gums are a symptom of leukaemia."

"Bleeding gums <u>are</u> a symptom of leukaemia," said Dr. King. "However, there are many other symptoms for that illness. Bleeding gums, without anything else, are highly unlikely to indicate a serious problem."

"Can you be sure?" Charlie asked.

"Well," answered Dr. King, "thousands of people suffer with bleeding gums, yet very few, a tiny proportion, have leukaemia."

"What could it be?" Charlie asked.

"At a guess," replied Dr. King, "gingivitis."

"What's that?" Charlie asked.

"Gum disease," replied the doctor, "nothing serious. Just ask your dentist when you next see him."

"Okay," said Charlie.

"You see," said Dr. King, "millions of people have bleeding gums but are in very good health."

"I appreciate that," answered Charlie, "but I always fear the worst. I just can't help it."

"Okay," said Dr. King, "this is what we'll do. During the week, if you get concerns regarding a serious ailment, write down the details. At your next appointment we can check the list and decide if you have anything to worry about."

"Thanks," said Charlie, "I'll do that."

Charlie wandered around the car park looking for his mother's vehicle.

"At least I can discuss all my health worries with Dr. King," he pondered. "So, I'll only have to worry about each problem 'til my next appointment. It won't stop me worrying completely but it'll be a great safety net."

Hazel's car was parked in the far corner next to a rusty death-trap that had definitely seen better times.

"Alright," said Charlie, opening the door, "let's go home."

Chapter 7

Time flew. Weeks turned into months. Worries were removed, then replaced.

It was a rainy Tuesday morning. Charlie and Charlotte watched as Hazel scrubbed the kitchen floor.

"Day off work," moaned Hazel, "I'd have more fun at the factory."

The phone shrilled, providing a welcome distraction.

"I'll get it," said Charlie, springing to his feet.

He almost flattened Hazel, such was his haste to answer the phone.

"Hello," he said.

"Hello, is that Charlie?"

"Yeah."

"It's William. Sorry I haven't been in touch for ages - relationships and work."

"Hello, Bill," said Charlie, "how are you?"

"Much the same," replied William, "except I've moved back with the folks. Still managing the cycle shop."

"Happy?" Charlie asked.

"Yes," answered William, "and what about you?"

"I'm okay," replied Charlie, "struggling on. Spend most of my time looking after Charlotte."

"Well," said William, "are you free this evening? We could go for a drink and a chat."

"Great," replied Charlie, "my mum will be able to look after Charlotte."

"Okay," said William, "I'll collect you about seven."

Charlie enjoyed a peaceful day with Charlotte and Hazel. He had a bath before going out.

"Hope tonight will be okay," he pondered, "if I get an irrational thought about being ill then I'm going to find it very difficult."

He climbed out the bath and grabbed the nearest towel.

"If I'm worrying, then I can't concentrate on anything else," he mused. "Not only will I have a terrible evening, but I'll also look a total space cadet."

He pulled on a black jumper and a clean pair of dungarees.

"Too late now," he decided, "Bill will be here in a few minutes."

William pulled up outside the house at a few minutes after seven.

"Bye," said Charlie, opening the door, "hope Charlotte doesn't wake up."

"She'll be fine," said Hazel, "try and have a good time."

Charlie climbed into the passenger seat.

"Hello, Bill," he said, "what are the plans?"

"There's a quiet pub in Clandon," answered William, "where we can have a drink and a chat."

"Fine," said Charlie.

William drove carefully, not once breaking the speed limit.

"You're looking trendy," said Charlie, "those clothes look really cool."

"Well," replied William, "have to look smart for work, but I hate wearing suits."

"What happened to the spikey hair?" Charlie asked.

"I got older," replied William, "had to have a suitable haircut for work."

Twenty-five minutes and they were parked outside The Bull's Head.

"Quaint," thought Charlie, "a nice, quiet pub. Ideal for a peaceful evening. Shouldn't be any drunken hooligans. Probably no graffiti in the toilets."

Charlie and William walked into the warm, dimly-lit bar. There were a few people scattered throughout the room. Two gentlemen stood at the bar. Smartly dressed, each sipping from a wine glass.

"Expect to see them in a library," pondered Charlie.

A young couple sat at a table by a large window. The young man, jeans and shirt, dark, shoulder-length hair, probably early twenties, kept touching the girl's hand across the table. She moved her hand as if electrocuted.

"Probably hoping to get his pecker felt," thought Charlie, "don't reckon he'll get lucky. At least, not with her."

An elderly couple sat by the entrance. The gentleman, at least eighty, nursed a half of bitter. The lady, roughly the same age, drank from a wine glass.

"It'll be okay," thought Charlie, breathing deeply, "there won't be a problem."

He gripped his dungaree straps and walked passed the

elderly couple. There wasn't an alternative route to the bar.

"No worries," thought Charlie, standing, with William, at the end of the bar.

William and Charlie chose a free table in the far corner of the room. William had a glass of cola; Charlie preferred lemonade.

"Didn't you fancy a beer?" Charlie asked.

"Never drink and drive," replied William, "not even one pint."

"Very wise," said Charlie.

Charlie rolled a cigarette.

"There's no way I'd have any alcohol," thought Charlie, "have to stay completely in control. And I'm not supposed to drink while I'm taking my medication."

William gulped a mouthful of cola.

"So, how's life with you?" Charlie asked.

"Well," replied William, "do you remember Sandra? Met her at the squash club. We were engaged for a while."

"Vaguely," replied Charlie.

"She broke off the engagement," continued William, "something about not pulling in the same direction."

"Oh," said Charlie. "When was this?"

"About three weeks ago," answered William.

"Were you gutted?" Charlie asked.

"At first," replied William, "I was devastated. Couldn't imagine carrying on without her. Wasn't eating or sleeping. I spent ages at work just to stop me thinking about her."

"Oh," said Charlie.

"But now," continued William, "I'm starting to come to terms with it. I'm young, free and single. Just want to have a good time."

Charlie picked up their two glasses from the table.

"Same again?" he asked.

"Lovely," answered William.

Charlie returned from the bar and plonked the drinks on the table.

"You look pleased with yourself," he said to William.

"Look over there," replied William, "by the fruit machine."

"Yeah," said Charlie, "two tarts. So what?"

"They're alone," said William, "we're alone……"

"Look," said Charlie, "ain't been interested in pulling since Linda. Got a child to consider."

"Just a friendly chat," said William, "where's the harm?"

"They look quite respectable," answered Charlie, eyeing the targets. "Doubt it'll be half a lager, packet of nuts and into the car park."

"Social interaction," said William, "is just as rewarding as a quick fumble outside the pub."

"If you say so," answered Charlie
.

Charlie and William stood near a table by the fruit machine.

"Okay if we sit here?" William asked, pointing at two empty seats.

"Okay," replied the taller girl.

"So what's the attraction of this pub?" William asked. "It's not very lively."

"Just fancied a quiet night."

"What are your names?" William asked.

"I'm Stacey and this is Catherine."

"I'm Bill and …….."

"I'm Charlie," interrupted Charlie.

Charlie took a sip from his glass.

"What the hell am I supposed to talk about," he thought, "can't think of anything remotely interesting to say."

William rubbed his chin, scratched his head, then fiddled with his earring.

"Well," thought Charlie," at least he ain't got a clue either."

"Do you work?" Stacey asked.

"I'm manager of a cycle shop," answered William.

"What about you?" Stacey asked, looking at Charlie.

"I'm looking for a permanent position," said Charlie, "want to find something with prospects."

"Oh," said Stacey.

"What about you?" William asked.

"We look after children with special needs," replied Catherine.

"Blimey," said Charlie, "must be hard work."

"It is," said Catherine, tall and slim with dark hair and a petite nose, "some of them are very poorly."

"How bad?" Charlie asked.

"None of them are able to walk or talk," replied Catherine, "we just feed them, change them and try to give them some quality of life."

"Are they terminally ill?" Charlie asked.

"Some of them," answered Catherine.

"How long have you worked with the children?" asked Charlie.

"Nearly six years," replied Catherine, twiddling the little gold stud in her nose.

"I've often thought about getting my nose pierced," said Charlie, "but never got round to it."

"It doesn't hurt," answered Catherine, "but I do feel it often gives a bad impression."

"Oh," said Charlie.

William watched as Stacey sipped her wine and puffed a menthol cigarette. She was a tall girl with a well proportioned figure. Long auburn hair and nice complexion. Make-up could have been applied by an expert. Very well groomed.

"Are you happy working with the children?" William asked, looking at Stacey.

"Very," replied Stacey.

"Don't you want a career?" William asked.

"I'm very happy at the moment," answered Stacey, with a slight frown, "thank-you."

"Why the fuck did he say that," wondered Charlie, "what's it to do with him if she's got a career or strips in some seedy club?"

Charlie took a drag on his roll-up.

"I always wanted to be a nurse," said Catherine.

"Wow," said Charlie, "that'd would be an amazing job."

"I thought so," said Catherine.

"Blimey," pondered Charlie, "this is someone who takes an interest in illnesses. Since I have different complaints nearly every day....... wow."

Charlie crushed his roll-up in the ashtray.

"So," he asked, "why did you never become a nurse?"

"Well," answered Catherine, "I failed the entrance exam."

"Oh," said Charlie, "gutted."

"However hard I tried," said Catherine, "I just couldn't understand the maths. I had loads of extra tuition, but still failed."

"What a shame," said Charlie, "you might have pulled a doctor."

"Since I finished with my last boyfriend," said Catherine, "I haven't wanted to get involved."

"Oh," said Charlie, "how long ago did you break up?"

STEPHEN DRAKE

"A couple of years," answered Catherine.

Charlie rolled another cigarette.

"You've got to admit," he said, "doctors are incredible people."

"What do you mean?" Catherine asked.

"Well," replied Charlie, "they're intelligent…….. they give you a sense of security."

"Are you joking?" Catherine asked.

"No way," answered Charlie, "I'm totally serious."

"I've never really thought about it," said Catherine. "I suppose it's because my dad is a doctor."

"What?" Charlie spluttered.

"I promise you," said Catherine, "he's a GP."

"That's amazing," said Charlie.

"If you say so," answered Catherine.

Charlie turned on his seat to face William.

"Book the church," he whispered, "don't fancy a long engagement."

Charlie swivelled back towards the two girls.

"You are so lucky," he said to Catherine, "you never have to worry about being ill. You can just check with your dad."

"I suppose I could," answered Catherine, "never really given it much thought."

"Amazing," repeated Charlie.

"Not very good when I tried to bunk off school," said Catherine, "he always knew when I was lying."

William gulped his drink then put the empty glass on the table.

"Okay Charlie," he said, "we'd better go. I've got an early start in the morning."

"Okay," replied Charlie.

Charlie turned towards Catherine.

"It's now or never," he decided, "if I don't say anything now, I'll never know."

He picked up his tobacco from the table.

"Can I have your phone number?" Charlie asked. "I'll call to check you got back safely."

"Yes," answered Catherine, "I'll give you my home number, but I'm staying the night at Stacey's, so I'd better give you her number as well."

"Great," said Charlie, "I'll call later so I know you've got back."

Catherine scribbled two numbers on a tatty piece of paper

94

and handed it to Charlie.

"Speak later," said Charlie.

William and Charlie headed for the exit

.

"Fucking pucker," thought Charlie. "A good night: no worries and a phone number."

The car travelled carefully along the quiet roads.

"Reckon you've got a good chance with Catherine," said William.

"Have to wait and see," replied Charlie.

"Did you like her?" William asked.

"Very nice," said Charlie.

The car pulled up outside Charlie's house.

"Fancy a coffee?" Charlie asked.

"No thanks," said William, "busy day tomorrow."

"Okay," said Charlie, "I'll call you."

Charlie, as quietly as possible, crept into the house, made a drink, rolled a cigarette and sat by the phone.

He sat for ten minutes, drinking and smoking.

"Here goes," he thought, "no point hanging about."

He took the piece of paper from his pocket, grabbed the phone and dialled.

"Hello," he said, "it's Charlie."

"Hi," replied Catherine.

"Got home safely, then," said Charlie.

"Been back about five minutes," said Catherine.

"Where's Stacey?" Charlie asked.

"Oh, she's in the bathroom getting ready for bed," replied Catherine. "I think she's a bit fed up. She didn't say much on the way home."

"Oh," said Charlie. "Did she mention Bill?"

"Briefly," answered Catherine. "She said he was a dickhead."

"Oh," said Charlie.

"She thought he was full of himself," said Catherine.

"Oh," repeated Charlie.

There were no awkward silences. Charlie would have been happy to talk all through the night. An hour had passed.

"Have you got a favourite child at work?" Charlie asked.

"It's a boy called Sean," replied Catherine, "he's so sweet."

"Is he really unwell?" Charlie asked.

"He can't do anything for himself," answered Catherine, "and he's blind."

"Blimey," said Charlie, "we don't know how lucky we are."
Charlie noticed a tingling sensation in his fingers wrapped around the handset.
"Bloody pins and needles," he thought, transferring the phone to his other hand, "what a pain in the bum."
"Multiple sclerosis. You remember reading about it. Starts with loss of sensation or pins and needles."
"Sort it out," he panicked, "don't be so bloody stupid."
He shook his hand, trying to shake off the pins and needles. His heart pounded and his breathing became rapid and shallow.
"Bloody hell," urged Charlie, "get control."
He tried to breathe deeply.
"You could be paralysed. There's no point trying to pull anyone. And you won't be much use to Charlotte."
"Think logically," he thought. "Pins and needles does not mean that you've got MS."
He took a large gulp of air.
"Don't get in a state," he thought, "I'll write down what I'm worried about and ask Dr. King."
Another gulp of air.
"Charlie," said Catherine, "are you still there? Is everything okay?"
"Er...... yeah......sorry," said Charlie, taking a check on reality.
"Most of the children we look after," said Catherine, "are born with their conditions."
"And the rest?" Charlie asked.
"Some have been abused, some have had terrible accidents," answered Catherine.
"What about their parents?" Charlie asked.
"They just can't cope," replied Catherine, "lots of the parents do come and visit their children."

Charlie and Catherine chatted happily, unaware the call had been over two hours long.
"Would you like to meet again?" Charlie asked.
"That'd be nice," replied Catherine.
"There's a quiet pub not far from here," said Charlie.
"Fine," answered Catherine.
"Next Friday, seven thirty, The Cricketers," said Charlie.
"Fine," repeated Catherine.
Charlie replaced the receiver and crept to his bedroom.

"Life is looking good," he pondered, "could be the start of something."

He folded his dungarees and placed them neatly on a chair.

"Trouble is…… you could have MS."

"Fuck off," he cursed, "I'm going to check with Dr. King."

He lay on his bed staring into the darkness.

"I'll check my worries with Dr. King and then I can concentrate on leading a normal life. I'll take care of Charlotte and see what happens with Catherine."

He smiled into the darkness.

"Not much any doctor can do if you've got MS!"

Sleep would rescue him……. eventually!

Chapter 8

Weeks became months. MS became leukaemia again, then Buerger's disease again, then MS again. But, despite all this, Charlie and Catherine formed a bond, growing stronger daily. Their first proper date had formed a solid base for a relationship to develop. Charlotte adapted to the new situation and appeared happy and settled.

It was a gloomy Tuesday. Charlie sat in the car, desperate to keep a lid on his anxieties. Catherine drove in silence. The hospital wasn't far and Dr. King should already be there.
"You'll feel much better when you've seen Dr. King," said Catherine, breaking the silence, "he'll be able to put your mind at rest."
"I hope so," replied Charlie.
Silence, except the engine purring and a faint voice from the direction of the radio.
"Here we are," said Catherine, parking the car.

Ten minutes sitting in the waiting room seemed like a week.
"Hello," said Dr. King, "how have you been?"
"Been worried most of the week," replied Charlie, "'bout having MS."
"What makes you think that?" D. King asked.
"Started with pins and needles in my hand," answered Charlie.
"Oh," said Dr. King.
"I looked in the medical book and now I seem to have most of the symptoms."
"Such as?" Dr. King asked.
"Blurred vision," answered Charlie, "especially when I'm watching tv"
"I see," said the psychiatrist, "and does worrying about MS affect daily life?"
"Yes," replied Charlie.
"Stand up," said Dr. King, "now follow my finger with your eyes."
Dr. King moved his finger slowly across Charlie's visual field.
"Okay," said Dr. King, "now stretch out your arm, finger facing the ceiling and bring your finger to your nose."

Charlie did as instructed.

"Fine," said Dr. King.

The neurological examination was completed.

"I can't find a problem," concluded Dr. King.

"Are you sure?" Charlie asked.

"I'd stake my mortgage on it," replied Dr. King.

"Thank-you," said Charlie.

"Who's the lovely young lady in the waiting room?" Dr. King asked.

"Oh, I met her quite a while ago," replied Charlie, "her father is a doctor."

"Oh," said Dr. King, "have you met him?"

"Not yet," replied Charlie.

"Some advice," said Dr. King, "about meeting him."

"Oh, yeah?" asked Charlie.

"Don't," replied Dr. King, smiling.

"Oh," said Charlie.

"You know," said Dr. King, "many people have blurred vision but don't have MS."

"I do," answered Charlie, "just got to convince myself."

"Well," said Dr. King, "as far as I can tell, you are fine. In perfect condition."

"Thank-you," said Charlie.

"I'll see you next time," concluded Dr. King.

Charlie and Catherine headed for home. Relieved, almost excited, the conversation flowed.

"So, it was okay?" Catherine asked.

"Brilliant," replied Charlie, "Dr. King is such a lovely man."

"Do you reckon your mum and Charlotte are having a good time?" Catherine asked.

"Hope so, "answered Charlie, "glad she had a day off work."

The following morning, sunny and bright, Catherine and Charlie took Charlotte to the park.

"Work tomorrow," said Catherine, pushing the swing.

"Yeah," replied Charlie, "you've had your two days off, now three days at work."

"I don't mind," said Catherine, "I enjoy seeing the children."

They hadn't been home much longer than twenty minutes when there was a knock at the door.

"Hello Debbie," said Charlie, opening the door.

"Hi," said Debbie, "I'm on my way to the bakery for a job

interview. I'm a bit early, so I thought I'd come and see you."

"Great," said Charlie, "have you got time for a coffee?"

"Go on then," said Debbie.

Catherine, Charlie and Debbie sat at the kitchen table, drinking and smoking. Charlotte, perched on the sofa in the lounge, watched Jungle Book on video again.

"Do you reckon you'll get the job?" Charlie asked.

"Not sure," replied Debbie, "I've never been very good at maths, so that could be a problem."

Charlie took a swig of coffee. His tongue felt a tiny lump, no bigger than a spot, on the inside of his cheek."

"What's that?" he wondered.

"Probably mouth cancer. You'll have to have major surgery. Your face will be a mess. Charlotte won't be able to look at you."

"Relax," he told himself, "think rationally."

"You okay, Charlie?" Catherine asked.

"Yeah," replied Charlie, fighting a pounding heart and quick, shallow breathing.

"I'd better get going," said Debbie, "it won't look very good if I'm late."

"Okay," managed Charlie, "hope it goes well."

Debbie shut the door as she left.

"Are you sure you're okay," repeated Catherine, "you're very quiet."

"It's just...." started Charlie, "I've got a little lump on the inside of my cheek. Do you think it could be something serious?"

"I doubt it," said Catherine, "can I have a look?"

Charlie opened his mouth and indicated the offending lump.

"Looks like an ulcer to me," said Catherine, "I'm sure it's nothing to worry about. You can always show Dr. King next week."

"Can't wait 'til then," replied Charlie, "could you ask your dad?"

"I'll ask him what he thinks," replied Catherine, "but he won't be certain unless he sees it."

"Okay," said Charlie, "just describe it to him and ask what he reckons."

"Okay then," sighed Catherine, "I'll phone him."

Afterwards, Catherine replaced the receiver and walked back into the kitchen.

"He says it does sound like an ulcer," said Catherine, "and

A CRY FOR EVER

he doesn't think that it's anything to worry about."

A week later, on a sunny Wednesday, Charlie and Catherine were wondering what to do.
"Let's take Charlotte to see Bessie and Snip," Charlie suggested.
"Your mum's two ponies," confirmed Catherine, "are they still in the same field?"
"Yeah," answered Charlie, "mum still rents the same field. Think she must have got a good deal."
"Good idea," said Catherine.
"Do you want to go and see the ponies, Tiger?" Charlie asked.
"Yes," answered Charlotte, "I love Bessie and Snip."
"Okay," said Charlie, "I'll just get some carrots."
They fed and stroked the ponies for almost an hour.
"Tiger is always happy when we come here," said Charlie, leaning over the sturdy wooden gate.
"She seems to be," replied Catherine.
"You know what I'd like to do?" Charlie asked.
"What's that?" Catherine said.
"I'm going to save a small amount of money each week and, when I've got enough, buy Tiger a pony of her own."
"That's a good idea," replied Catherine.

Catherine had been working twelve hour shifts for the last three days. Tuesday was her first day off work, and Charlie was really pleased to see her. It was just after lunch and Charlie, Catherine and Charlotte were watching Jungle Book........ again.
Charlie stood-up and walked into the kitchen.
"Think we need to go to the supermarket," said Charlie, looking in the cupboards.
"Okay," said Catherine, "let's watch the end of the video and then we can go."

People hurried along the aisles. Charlie felt extreme anxiety watching the melee, and fought the urge to leave the shop.
"Come on," he urged himself, "you've got Catherine with you. This'll be easy."
Catherine found a trolley and the task begun.
"Lemonade," said Catherine, putting a bottle in the trolley.
"Crisps," said Charlie, grabbing a bag.

"Get some biscuits," said Catherine.

"Okay," replied Charlie, reaching for chocolate digestives.

"You hit an old lady. You've hurt her."

"Oh bollocks," panicked Charlie, checking that the nearby customers were all okay.

Five yards to his left, leaning over her trolley, with grey hair and a walking stick, hovered a defenceless old woman.

"Oh hell," thought Charlie, anxiety rising, "what have I done?"

He leaned against a stone pillar. His heart was in his mouth, and his stomach was in knots. Mouth dry and vision distorted.

He watched intently as the old lady put some doughnuts in her trolley.

"She's fine," he thought, "you haven't done anything."

"What if she's hurt and collapses somewhere else?"

"Don't be so dumb," he thought, fighting the doubts, "nothing happened."

"You okay, Charlie? Catherine asked.

"Er…….. yeah," he struggled.

"You look like you've seen a ghost," said Catherine.

"Did I do anything strange?" Charlie asked.

"How do you mean?" Catherine replied.

"Well," said Charlie, "did I just do anything that you might consider odd or offensive?"

"Nothing at all," replied Catherine.

"Are you absolutely sure?" Charlie pushed.

"Course I am," said Catherine, "don't you think that I'd have said something?"

Anxiety dropped. Charlie felt pardoned. He had fallen from the tight-rope but landed in the safety net.

They chatted during the short journey home.

"Think we got everything," said Catherine.

"I hope so," replied Charlie.

"You hit that old woman."

"Don't be silly," thought Charlie, anxiety rising, "you checked at the time."

"Are you okay?" Catherine asked.

"Yeah," replied Charlie.

"You're having a bad day," said Catherine.

"You remember when we were in the shop," said Charlie,"

and I asked if I'd done anything odd?"

"Yes," answered Catherine.

"Well," said Charlie, "are you absolutely certain?"

"Yes," said Catherine.

"You were watching me all the time?"

"Yes," repeated Catherine.

"You'd be prepared to swear to it in court?"

"I would," answered Catherine.

The safety-net didn't buckle under the strain.

Charlotte had just fallen asleep.

"Eight o'clock," thought Charlie, glancing at the clock, "not too late."

He walked into the lounge and slumped onto the sofa. Catherine was flicking through the channels trying to find a decent programme.

"What a day," said Charlie, "I'm knackered."

"Yes," replied Catherine, "and there doesn't seem to be much on television."

"What's that?" Charlie thought, noticing a mark on his hand.

It was a red spot. Quite large, deep red, but just a spot.

"That's how the superbug enters your body."

"Bloody hell," panicked Charlie, "what if I've got the superbug."

Charlie fidgeted on the sofa. His heart raced, his breathing became shallow and rapid. His vision blurred, head pounded. He wrestled with an urge to vomit.

"Shit," he panicked, "the little bugger could eat me alive."

Perspiration prickled on his forehead.

"Got to see a doctor," he decided, "it'll be too late to wait for my next appointment with Dr. King."

"What's the matter?" Catherine asked.

"Oh......... um ...."

"You look terrible," said Catherine, "really awful."

"I'm worried I've got the superbug," divulged Charlie, holding out his hand, "you know, the bug that's always in the papers."

"That's a spot," said Catherine, looking at his hand.

"The bug enters the skin and leaves a mark," said Charlie.

"Okay," said Catherine, patiently, "apart from that mark, do you feel okay?"

"Shitting myself," replied Charlie.

"Physically," said Catherine, "any other symptoms?"

"Nothing," answered Charlie.

"Well," said Catherine, "if the little bug had entered your system, you would be very ill. Terrible headache, raging sore throat, sky-high temperature."

"You sure?"

"You would be in a really bad way," answered Catherine, "try not to think about it."

"I'll try," said Charlie.

The evening passed, Charlie wasn't eaten alive, so his anxiety lowered.

The next day dawned, bright and sunny. Catherine, free from work, was spending time with Charlie and Charlotte.

Charlie and Catherine sat at the kitchen table, drinking coffee and smoking. Morning's nicotine fix- essential! Morning's caffeine fix - equally important! Charlotte sat in the lounge watching...... Jungle Book.

"Nice day," said Charlie, "shall we go to the park? Or do you fancy a walk in the woods?"

"Don't mind," answered Catherine.

"What would you like to do, Tiger?" Charlie asked.

"Don't mind," said Charlotte.

"Okay," said Charlie, "let's go to the park."

"Right," said Catherine.

"I'm just going to put some money in Tiger's pony pot," whispered Charlie to Catherine, "won't be a minute."

Charlie walked into Lucy's bedroom and opened the cupboard. Top shelf, Tiger's pony pot.

Charlie stuffed ten pounds into the pot.

"Must have quite a bit," he thought, "must count it when I've got a spare minute."

He went back to the kitchen.

"Ready?"

There was a knock on the door.

"Who would that be?" Charlie asked, walking to the door.

"Hello," said Julian, "long time, no see."

"Hello Julian," said Charlie, "what brings you here?"

"No work," replied Julian, "not much happening, so I thought I'd see how you were doing."

"We were going to the park," said Charlie, "but I suppose we can go later."

Julian sat at the table, chain smoking. It wasn't long before the ashtray was overflowing.

"Can I have a go on Lucy's computer?" Julian asked. "I want to finish 'Mario'."

"Okay," answered Charlie.

Julian walked into Lucy's bedroom, puffing on another cigarette.

Another knock on the door.

"Blimey," thought Charlie, heading for the door, " who's here now?"

Debbie and Anna were at the door.

"Thought we'd come and visit," said Anna.

"Oh, right," said Charlie.

"Guess the park will still be around tomorrow," he thought.

The following day, again bright and sunny. Charlie, Catherine and Charlotte were getting ready for a day at the park. There was a knock on the door. Charlie opened the door. Richard and Edward this time.

"Hello, Charlie," said Edward, "time for a coffee?"

"Guess so," sighed Charlie, "by the time we get Charlotte to the park, she'll be able to go on her own."

Six cups of coffee, twenty roll-ups, and two toasted cheese sandwiches later:

"I'd better get going," said Richard, "got to change the brakes on my van."

"Okay," said Charlie, " see you soon."

"I'll just have one more coffee," said Edward, rolling a cigarette, "then I'd better get going as well."

The following day, and not a visitor in sight. It rained steadily.

"No park, today," said Charlie, "how about 'Crazy Tots' at the leisure centre?"

Days became weeks. Visitors were in steady supply. Apart from her time at work, Catherine practically lived with Charlie and Charlotte. Illnesses caused concern with varying levels of anxiety.

It was a gorgeous Wednesday afternoon. Charlie, Catherine and Charlotte had just enjoyed a trip to the park.

"Perfect day for it," said Charlie, making Charlotte a drink.

"Really good," agreed Catherine.

The kettle boiled.

"Really fancy a coffee," said Catherine.

There was a knock on the door.

"Another visitor," thought Charlie, opening the door.

"Hi," said Trudy, "hope you don't mind me popping round."

"Not at all," said Charlie, "come in. Catherine and Charlotte are here."

Trudy only lived a short walk from Charlie, but appeared breathless. She was a very pretty girl, couple of years older than Charlie, quick sense of humour and heavy smoker.

"You've had your hair chopped off," said Charlie.

"I've had it cut into a bob," said Trudy, " and bleached."

"How's work?" Charlie asked.

"Good," replied Trudy, "but the boss, who's well over sixty, keeps patting my bum."

"Oh," said Charlie, "and you're not keen?"

"He's hardly Edward," answered Trudy.

"What about pay?" Charlie asked.

"Not enough," replied Trudy, "barely keeps me in fags."

They chatted, drank coffee and smoked.

"Bloody hell," pondered Charlie, as Trudy lit another cigarette from the last, "she'd need to be a brain surgeon to keep her in fags."

Days passed, weather stayed fine, fear of illness kept reappearing, safety-net did its job. It was a Monday afternoon. The morning had been spent trudging through the woods. Charlotte was tired, so a video was the perfect answer. Charlie and Catherine tried to feign enthusiasm as Jungle Book blared from the corner of the room.

"I think I'll go and count the money in the pot," said Charlie, "it must be nearly one hundred pounds."

He walked into Lucy's room and took the pot from the cupboard.

"Thirty pounds," he said, holding the notes, "what the fuck's going on?"

He checked his sums.

"Two tens and two fives," he said, "what's happening here? There should be about a hundred quid."

He checked, just to be sure the pot was empty.

"I've been robbed," he cursed, "some bastard has nicked Tiger's money."

He hurried back into the kitchen.

"Cath," he said, "guess what?"

106

"What?" Catherine asked.

"Some fucker has nicked the money I've been saving."

"What, all of it?"

"There's only thirty quid left in the pot," said Charlie, "at least sixty quid has gone."

"Who would do something like that?" Catherine said.

"Suppose it could be anyone," replied Charlie, "so many people come here and wander into Lucy's room."

"I can't believe anyone would steal from the house," said Catherine.

"Well," said Charlie, "somebody definitely has."

"What can we do?" Catherine asked.

"Not sure," replied Charlie.

"What about the police?"

"Don't think so," answered Charlie.

"What then?"

"We'll have to play it carefully," replied Charlie, "take our time, keep checking the money in the pot, then we can work out what to do."

"Wouldn't it be better to hide the rest of the money?" Catherine suggested.

"Then we'll never find out who nicked the sixty quid," answered Charlie. "We need to know who has been robbing. It's Tiger's money so……. I need to know."

"Okay," agreed Catherine.

Over the next few days, many visitors filed through the house. Some stayed for ages, others less than an hour. Some went into Lucy's room, others didn't. Some might have, although Charlie wasn't watching all the time. It was a Monday night, after nine, and Charlotte had finally dropped off.

"Come on," said Charlie to Catherine, "let's check the pot."

"Okay," sighed Catherine, "but I don't think you'll find anything missing."

"Soon see," replied Charlie, heading for Lucy's room.

Charlie took the pot from the cupboard. Catherine watched as he handled the notes.

"Shit," he cursed, "I don't fucking believe it."

"What?"

"Another ten has gone," said Charlie.

"Are you sure?"

"Positive," answered Charlie, "there are two fives and one

ten."

"And you're sure there were two tens?"

"I'd stake my life on it," answered Charlie.

"What are you thinking?" Catherine asked.

"Well," replied Charlie, "we've got to work out who's had the opportunity to take the money."

"Okay," said Catherine.

"Let's go and have a coffee," said Charlie, "and talk it over."

They talked, smoked and drank coffee for the next hour. Lucy came home from the pub, had a quick drink, then went to bed. Hazel arrived within a few minutes, having spent the evening with a friend.

"Goodnight," said Hazel, heading for bed, "try and keep the noise down."

"Okay," replied Charlie, "goodnight."

Another coffee, more nicotine and plenty of chat. It was gone midnight.

"So," said Charlie, "you agree that only four people had the opportunity."

"Well," replied Catherine, "I can't be sure, but it looks that way."

"Right," said Charlie, "we've got a list of possible suspects."

"Suppose," answered Catherine.

"Trudy, Julian, Anna and Debbie," said Charlie.

"That's what I reckon," replied Catherine.

"Okay," said Charlie. "Now, we've got to cut the list to one."

"And how do you suggest we do that?"

"Leave the pot in the same place, act normally, keep checking the money and keep a close eye on the famous four."

"Right," said Catherine, "I'm exhausted. I'm going to bed."

Days passed. People continued to come and go. The famous four were regular visitors. No more money went missing.

Saturday afternoon, and the rain lashed against the kitchen window. Charlotte was with her mother. Catherine had a twelve hour shift at work. Charlie sat at the kitchen table, drinking coffee, smoking and chatting to Julian.

"So," said Charlie, " you had a good week?"

"Not bad," answered Julian, "bit boring, but okay."

"I've had a busy week," said Charlie, "looking after Charlotte can be quite tiring."

"Yeah," said Julian, "reckon she can be a bit of a brat."

Charlie swigged his coffee and puffed his roll-up.

"Look," he said, "I'm going to have a bath, so you'd better get going."

"Okay," said Julian, "see you later."

Julian closed the door as he left. Charlie paced the kitchen floor.

"Who the fuck is he," cursed Charlie, "to talk like that about Charlotte?"

He sat at the table and rolled a cigarette.

"I reckon it was him," pondered Charlie. "I think Julian nicked the money."

He stood up, flicked the kettle switch and waited.

"Got to be him," he decided, "probably spent all Tiger's money on booze. She won't get a pony but, who cares, Julian can get pissed."

Charlie was building a case on evidence so circumstantial and flimsy, it hardly existed.

"Yeah," he concluded, "Julian robbed the money and spent it down the pub."

The case had been heard. The jury had reached a verdict. Guilty. Now, all that had to be done was to pass sentence.

Charlie spent the day smoking and drinking. As he puffed and slurped, he mused on his current problem.

"Got to do something," he thought, for the thousandth time, "can't let the fucker get away with it. Then again, don't want to be arrested cause I need to be here for Charlotte."

That evening, just after nine, Charlie phoned Catherine. She shared a house with two health workers and stayed at home when she had work the following day.

"Hi," said Charlie, "it's me."

"Hi," said Catherine, "how are you?"

"Good," replied Charlie, "spent the day thinking."

"Oh," said Catherine.

"I'm pretty sure I know who nicked the money," said Charlie.

"Who?"

"Julian," replied Charlie.

"How do you know?"

"Worked it out. Brains. It has to be him," lied Charlie.

"Oh," repeated Catherine.

"I'm sure," lied Charlie.

"So, what now?"

"Well," answered Charlie, "I've been thinking about it all day."

"And?"

"I've got a plan," said Charlie.

"Which is?"

"Have you got a friend who owes you a favour?"

"I could find someone," answered Catherine, "there's a care assistant called Michaela. She'll help. Depending on what it is."

"When I tell you," said Charlie, "could you ask her to phone Julian? He definitely won't recognise her voice. Tell him that I've shown her a photo of him and she reckons he's a bit hunky."

"Why?"

"Well," continued Charlie, swept along with the plan, "get her to ask him for a drink in the pub. It has to be The Crown."

"Hold on," said Catherine, "she won't go and meet Julian."

"She hasn't got to," replied Charlie. "she just has to arrange a date in The Crown. I know the way he'll go to the pub and I can talk to him then."

"What are you going to do?"

"Nothing for you to worry about," replied Charlie. "Do you think she'll help?"

"I suppose so," sighed Catherine, "I'll ask her tomorrow."

"Thanks," said Charlie.

They had been on the phone for nearly three hours.

"Suppose I'd better go," said Catherine, "early start in the morning."

"Okay," answered Charlie, "please ask Michaela and I'll phone you tomorrow."

Charlie lazed around the house most of Sunday. Nothing on television, no good books, Charlotte at Linda's and Catherine at work. He lay on his bed staring at the ceiling.

"Got to get Julian sorted," he pondered, "hope Catherine's friend will help."

The day trudged by. He looked at the clock – it was a few minutes after nine o'clock.

"Good," he thought, "Catherine will be home from work."

He made a coffee, rolled a cigarette and settled by the phone.

A CRY FOR EVER

"Hi," said Charlie, "good day at work?"

"Not too bad," answered Catherine.

"Did you get a chance to talk to Michaela?"

"I did," replied Catherine.

"And?"

"She'll phone him," said Catherine.

"Great," enthused Charlie.

"She was a bit confused," said Catherine.

"What did you tell her?"

"I was very vague," answered Catherine, "just implied it was going to be a joke."

"That's fine," said Charlie.

They chatted for over two hours.

"See you on Wednesday," said Charlie.

"Yes," agreed Catherine, "see you then."

Tuesday arrived, hot and sunny. Charlie and Charlotte came back from the park gasping for a drink.

"Put a video on, Tiger," said Charlie, "I'm just going to make a quick call."

"Hello," said Charlie.

"Oh, hello," replied Julian.

"Are you busy?" Charlie asked.

"No," answered Julian, "just sitting about."

"Want to pop round?"

"Yeah," replied Julian, "see you soon."

Charlie and Julian sat at the kitchen table, drinking and smoking. Charlotte lay on the sofa watching Jungle Book.

"I've got something to show you," said Charlie.

"What's that?" Julian replied.

"Hold on a minute," answered Charlie.

He hurried to his room, opened a drawer and took out a photo.

"Glad I kept this picture," thought Charlie, "Jane's friend. Think her name was Fran."

He walked back into the kitchen.

"Take a look," said Charlie, handing the photo to Julian.

Julian stared at the picture. A very attractive young lady. Quite tall with a slim and well-proportioned figure. Very pretty face and dark hair, beautifully styled in a short cut. Her glasses added to her appearance, suggesting an intelligent, successful person. Her smart clothes reinforced this idea.

"So?" said Julian.

"What do you think?" Charlie asked.

"I've seen worse," replied Julian.

"She's gorgeous," said Charlie.

"So what? Who is she?"

"Well," answered Charlie, "she's a friend of Jane's."

"And?"

"She wants to meet you," said Charlie.

"Fuck off," said Julian, "she doesn't even know me."

"Well," said Charlie, "Jane showed her a photo of you."

"Why?"

"Well," answered Charlie, "we thought you might like some action."

"Oh, did you?"

"Yeah," said Charlie, "just park and ride."

"You're taking the piss," said Julian.

"Truthfully," said Charlie, "I'm not lying. She likes you."

"I'm not sure."

"Look," said Charlie, "I'll ask Jane to get her to phone you."

"Okay," answered Julian, "we'll see."

They chatted for the next few hours. Plenty of caffeine, and Julian had enough nicotine to kill an ox.

"Better get going," said Julian.

"Okay," replied Charlie, "can I tell Jane you're interested in her mate?"

"Suppose," replied Julian.

"I'll get her to give you a buzz," said Charlie.

"Okay," said Julian.

"Just remember," said Charlie, "play safe and keep it legal."

"Piss off," answered Julian, leaving the house.

Charlie found Catherine's phone number at work. He tried not to phone while she was working, but in an emergency...........

"Hi," said Charlie.

"Oh, hello," replied Catherine.

"Is Michaela at work today?"

"She is," replied Catherine.

"Can you get her to phone Julian? Arrange to meet at The Crown. Let me know when; the sooner the better."

"Okay," sighed Catherine, "I'll ask her now. I'll phone you as soon as she's spoken to him."

Charlie relayed Julian's phone number to her. Catherine wrote it down carefully.

He paced the kitchen.

"Want to get this sorted," he pondered, "as soon as possible."

"To be honest, you're not sure that Julian took the money!"

Charlie slumped at the kitchen table. Charlotte dozed peacefully on the sofa.

"I reckon he did," he thought, dismissing a massive doubt, "I hope he did. Anyway, he called Tiger a brat."

He stood up and paced.

"What if you're making an awful mistake. You've no proof. You're just guessing."

"Bollocks," he muttered, "I can't just forget about it."

The phone rang. Charlie hurried into the lounge, not wanting Charlotte to be disturbed.

"Hi," he said.

"Hi," said Catherine, "she's arranged to meet him at The Crown at eight o'clock this evening."

"Bloody hell," said Charlie, "he doesn't hang about."

"Don't do anything stupid," warned Catherine, "see you tomorrow."

"Okay," replied Charlie, "thanks."

Charlotte stirred on the sofa. She rubbed her eyes and sat up.

"Morning, Tiger," said Charlie, "I'll make you some breakfast."

Charlotte ate a marmite sandwich and drank blackcurrant as Mr. Blobby danced on the video. A break from Jungle Book....... at last!

Charlie phoned Anna. He wasn't sure why..... just wanted to talk.

"Hi," said Anna.

"Hello," replied Charlie.

They had been chatting for about fifteen minutes. Mr. Blobby continued to dance on screen.

"Going to jump out at Julian this evening," said Charlie, "he's meeting a bird in the pub and I'm going to wait for him."

"What you going to do?" Anna asked.

"Not sure," replied Charlie, "but I think he's stolen money from me."

"Are you sure?" Anna asked.

"Well……… um…………….."

"You're not sure, are you?"

"Not exactly," admitted Charlie.

"Just don't do anything you might regret," sighed Anna.

"Okay," said Charlie, "Speak to you soon."

Charlie paced the kitchen, smoked a roll-up and gulped a coffee. Then he phoned Debbie and had a similar conversation. Then he phoned Trudy. Again the conversation followed a familiar line. Edward's opinion was much the same.

Charlie and Charlotte watched Jungle Book, drew some pictures and danced to music. Then, Charlie sipped a well-earned coffee while Charlotte watched Jungle Book again - just in case she'd forgotten the end.

"Hope tonight goes to plan," pondered Charlie, "what if something goes wrong?"

"What if you hit an old woman instead of Julian."

"That ain't gonna happen," thought Charlie, "I doubt any old ladies will be wandering along dark alleys that time of the evening."

"How can you be so sure."

Charlie rolled a cigarette.

"Okay," he decided, "I'll take someone with me. Then I'll be able to check."

He finished his roll-up, stood up and walked to the phone.

"Hello," said Charlie.

"Hi," said Richard, "how are you?"

"Not too bad," replied Charlie, "but I could do with a favour."

"What's that?"

"Well," answered Charlie, "are you free this evening?"

"Yeah," replied Richard.

"Could you meet me in Fetcham at the end of dog-shit alley?"

"Why?" Richard asked.

"Something I need to do," replied Charlie.

"You're not robbing, are you?"

"No," answered Charlie.

"What then?"

"Look," answered Charlie, "I know that Julian is going to The Crown tonight. The best way is along dog-shit alley. I want to meet him for a little chat."

114

A CRY FOR EVER

"Nothing dodgy?" Richard asked.

"Hope not," answered Charlie.

"What's he done?" Richard asked.

"I think he stole some money from me," replied Charlie.

"Are you sure?"

"Almost," lied Charlie.

"Oh, okay," said Richard, "what time?"

"Seven thirty," answered Charlie.

"Okay," said Richard, "I'll be there."

The rest of the day passed in a blur. Lucy came home from work after six. Problems at the office, apparently.

"Hi," said Charlie.

"Hello," replied Lucy, "I'm exhausted."

"Oh," said Charlie, "I was wondering if you'd keep an eye on Charlotte tonight."

"Suppose so," replied Lucy, "too tired to go out."

"Great," enthused Charlie.

"What are you doing?"

"Nothing much," answered Charlie, "just meeting up with somebody."

It was almost six-thirty. Charlie searched, frantically, in a cupboard in the garage.

"Here it is," he said, pulling out a balaclava, "thank fuck."

He took a pair of gardening gloves from the top of the cupboard and went back into the house.

It was quarter to seven. He took his jacket from the peg, put his knife in his pocket and headed into the night.

"No way will I use the knife," he thought, "but I always carry it."

He walked on.

"Hang on," he thought, "if I get nicked and they find a knife I'll be fucked."

He hurried home and put the knife in the garage. Balaclava and gloves tucked in his jacket, Charlie set off.

"Hope Richard turns up," he pondered, hurrying through the darkness.

Twenty past seven, and he was nearly there.

"Just get tonight sorted," he pondered, "and then carry on looking after Charlotte."

Charlie arrived ahead of schedule. Dogshit alley was dirty, dark and well- hidden.

"This'll be perfect," he decided.

Richard, reliability faultless, arrived within ten minutes of his friend. He was limping heavily.

"Hello," said Charlie.

"Hi," said Richard."

"What's wrong with your leg?" Charlie asked.

"It's my fucking foot," answered Richard, "it's killing me. I've been having a lot of trouble with it over the last few months."

"You'll be okay, though?"

"Yeah," answered Richard, "I can walk, but it's one hell of a struggle."

"Okay," said Charlie," let's walk down the alley and find a place we can hide. Don't want Julian to see us and get away."

"What do you want to do?"

"Just talk to him."

"So," asked Richard, pointing at Charlie's pocket, "why have you got a balaclava and gloves?"

"Well," replied Charlie, "best be prepared."

"Yeah," sighed Richard.

They walked along the alley, avoiding piles of dogshit, looking for a hideout.

"Got to be somewhere we'll be able to stay hidden 'til he's close enough," said Charlie.

"Okay," sighed Richard.

They found a hidden turning halfway along the alley.

"No street lights," said Charlie, "pitch dark. Perfect."

They stood in position, chilled by the night air, and waited.

"How do you know that Julian's going to The Crown?" Richard asked.

"He's got a date," replied Charlie, "and I reckon he'll be shagged."

"Yeah," sighed Richard, "who'd give up a chance for a romp with Julian."

Charlie put his balaclava on his head, leaving his face uncovered. The gardening gloves did little to protect his hands from the cold.

"Look," said Richard, "my foot is fucking agony. I'm gonna have to sit down."

"Bit cold," answered Charlie.

"I know," said Richard, "but I can't take the pain in my foot."

A CRY FOR EVER

Richard sat on the pavement, legs outstretched. Charlie stood, out of sight, listening intently.

"He's got to be here soon," thought Charlie, "he won't be able to resist the chance of a shag."

Footsteps in the distance.

"Hang on," said Charlie, "I think he's coming."

Richard didn't reply. He sat on the floor, wincing in pain, holding his foot. Charlie listened, hardly daring to breathe. The footsteps grew louder. Charlie peered from his hidden location. Julian pounded along the alley, breathing heavily.

"If he didn't smoke so much and lost a bit of weight," pondered Charlie, "a ten minute stroll wouldn't seem like a marathon."

Julian was within five yards. Charlie's unsteady gloved hand pulled the balaclava over his face.

"Now I've come this far," decided Charlie, "got to follow it through."

He stepped out of hiding and stood in front of Julian. Julian stopped walking. Silence, except for gasping breaths. Charlie's gloved right hand landed perfectly. A winning smash in tennis or a hole-in-one in golf.

"Felt like teeth," thought Charlie, "that'll do."

Julian sank to the pathway. Hands instinctively covering his head. Legs lifted to his stomach making the smallest possible target.

"Got to give him a bit more," thought Charlie, "started so might as well finish."

Adrenalin pumping, Charlie darted across the alley. He aimed blow after blow at Julian's head. Limited visibility and Julian's hands prevented lasting damage. Julian groaned as each gloved punch connected.

"Can't really see what state he's in," thought Charlie, "so dark, can't even see if he's bleeding."

One last punch, the thud of skull on pavement, and Charlie straightened up from his crouched position. A kick, aimed at Julian's crumpled body, satisfied the assailant.

"Come on," shouted Charlie to Richard, pocketing balaclava and gloves, "let's go."

Richard struggled to his feet and limped along the alley. Charlie trotted beside his friend, desperate to distance himself from the scene.

"What if you got the wrong man? He might not have taken

the money. What if he dies? He looked in a bad way."

Charlie and Richard left the alley, passed the shops and reached a local estate.

"I'm sure he'll be fine," thought Charlie, "nothing too serious."

"What if he didn't take the money?"

Richard limped down the estate, pain etched on his face. Charlie, jogging slowly, struggled to keep a grip on his anxiety.

"You wanted to do it," he thought, "now live with what you've done."

They were a few hundred yards from the end of the estate. Richard slowed, then stopped.

"My foot," he moaned, "need a rest."

"Once we get to the end of this road," said Charlie, "we should be okay."

"Stop. Police!"

"Fuck," said Charlie, looking around, "oh, fuck."

A plain-clothed detective, waving a warrant card, headed towards the two men. Other police seemed to appear from thin air. Two cars skidded to a halt, closely followed by a van, loaded with uniformed officers.

"Shit," said Richard, "they're fucking everywhere. We've been followed from the alley. Somebody grassed us."

The detective, big and bulky with cropped hair and scarred face, took a firm hold of each man.

"You're under arrest for robbery," he said.

"Robbery?" Charlie repeated.

"You're nicked, sonny."

It was a matter of seconds before Charlie and Richard were surrounded. Charlie was stood against one car while Richard was led to the other. A young constable, promotion in mind, searched Charlie's pockets. He pulled out the balaclava and gloves.

"Oh dear," he said, displaying the items, "you're in trouble."

Dorking police station hadn't changed. The custody suite was just as Charlie remembered. He sat in the cell, struggling to concentrate, consumed with self-pity and regret.

"What the fuck have I done?"

He stood up and paced the miserable cell. Same as ever. Wooden bench, ripped blue mattress, filthy grey blanket, dirty walls covered in obscenities, not forgetting the disgusting toilet in desperate need of a good scrub.

"I could get put away for this," panicked Charlie, "won't be much use to Tiger in prison. What if they refuse bail? I won't have a chance to make any arrangements. Oh, bollocks!"

He sat on the bench, head in hands.

"Even worse," he pondered, anxiety sky high, "what if Julian is badly hurt or dies......... oh, fuck me."

A few more lengths of the cell.

"And," he thought, "what if Julian didn't take the money. I've done all this for fuck all."

Charlie quickened his pace.

"So," he thought, "in summary, the worse case scenario is that I could be looking at years away from Tiger. And Julian could be badly hurt, or worse, for something he didn't even do."

He leaned against the wall.

"Look," he urged, "for fuck's sake, think clearly. You've got yourself in this situation, now...... what's the best way out of it?"

He paced the cell. The prison walk. Never get anywhere and bloody boring.

"If I deny it," he pondered, "have they got enough to charge me? They were in the alley, but did they see exactly what happened? Could they identify me as the person who hit Julian?"

The cell door opened, interrupting Charlie's defence preparations. The lanky jailer, near retirement age, stood in the doorway.

"Lloyd interview. Come with me."

Charlie was shown to the first interview room.

"I'm DS Keen," said the detective, short, fat and female with dark, curly hair, a big nose, squinty eyes and a slight facial hair problem. "We have spoken to Julian at the hospital and realise the offence we are investigating is assault rather than robbery."

Sitting next to DS Keen was DC Thorpe, a tall man, smartly dressed, tidy haircut and boyish good looks.

How's Julian?" Charlie asked.

"He's lost a few teeth," replied the officer, "but he'll live."

"Thank fuck," thought Charlie.

"So," began DS Keen, "what had you been doing when you

were arrested?"

"No comment," replied Charlie.

"Why were you carrying a balaclava?"

"No comment," replied Charlie.

A few more questions went unanswered.

"Right," said DS Keen, "we're getting nowhere. You're going back to your cell but I want you to have a little think. If you fail to answer any questions we will have to investigate further. We will look into the phone call to Julian."

"Phone call?" Charlie repeated.

"Yes," said DS Keen," we've got the facts from Julian."

"Oh," said Charlie.

"We'll have to trace the person who made that call."

"Oh," said Charlie.

"Okay," concluded DS Keen, " have a little think about it."

Afterwards, Charlie perched on the bench and contemplated his best move.

"Don't want anyone else involved," he pondered, "I'm to blame."

He sat back against the wall.

"I'd better admit it and pray for a lenient magistrate," he decided, "can't risk anyone else getting nicked."

He stood up and paced.

"Shouldn't get long," he thought. "Julian only lost a few teeth. Might even get a bit more probation. Just hope I get bailed 'til my case. Then I can get Tiger sorted."

He banged on the cell door.

"Hold on," shouted the jailer, "be with you in a minute."

Charlie stood by the door staring at the hatch. Seconds later, the hatch opened and a face appeared.

"What?"

"Ready for another interview," said Charlie, "got something to say."

"Okay."

DS Keen and DC Thorpe sat at the table. Charlie fidgeted on his chair, drummed his fingers, and studied, with exaggerated interest, the patterned carpet.

"Okay," began DS Keen, "you asked to speak to us."

"Yeah," blurted Charlie, "it was me."

"Right," said DS Keen, "would you like to put your side of events?"

A CRY FOR EVER

Charlie recounted the night's events.

"So," said DS Keen, "was Richard involved? He hasn't answered any questions."

"He didn't know what was going to happen," answered Charlie, "and he wasn't involved at all."

"Okay," said DC Thorpe.

"He speaks," thought Charlie, "he's not just arm candy."

"Why did you do it?" DS Keen asked.

"Um......."

"It's very rare for an attack to be unprovoked," she continued. "Julian didn't know why he was targeted."

"I think he took some money from my house," muttered Charlie.

"Do you wish to make a complaint?"

"No," replied Charlie, "no proof."

"Okay," concluded DS Keen, "interview terminated."

Charlie sat in his cell for nearly two hours. Finally, he was taken to the custody suite and stood before the desk sergeant. He remembered the drill.

"You are charged with assaulting Julian Mason, occasioning actual bodily harm on..................."

Charlie's mind started to wander.

"Hope Tiger is okay with Lucy," he thought, "and hope Catherine's not too worried."

"Do you understand the charge?"

"Yeah," replied Charlie.

"Do you have anything to say?"

"No," he replied.

"You will be bailed to appear at Dorking Magistrates' Court on.........."

Charlie left the police station. Richard was waiting outside. A CID officer drove the young men back home.

Seven days became a week. Court loomed like a dark cloud in the distance. Charlie and Catherine sat at the table, taking in caffeine and nicotine. Charlotte lay on the sofa watching Mr. Blobby.

"Only a few more days 'til court," said Charlie.

"Yes," replied Catherine, "what do you reckon will happen?"

"They could fine me, I suppose," said Charlie, "but most likely they'll ask for pre-sentence reports. That shouldn't take long 'cause I'm already seeing Mr. Carson."

"What do you think he'll recommend?"

"Wouldn't like to say," answered Charlie, "custody or more probation."

A trip to the park was interrupted by a downfall of rain. Back home, they drew some pictures as Jungle Book played in the background. Charlie and Catherine went into the kitchen; it had been nearly two hours since their last cup of coffee. They sat at the table, sipping, chatting and smoking.

"What's going to happen with Charlotte," said Catherine, "if the worst does happen when you go to court."

"I'll have to talk to Linda," answered Charlie, "they'll both be fine. Tiger is always happy when she goes to see Linda at the weekends."

The following day, Catherine and Charlie took Charlotte to the leisure centre. 'Crazy Tots' was on the agenda. Back home, after lunch, Charlie phoned Linda.

"Hello," he said.

"Oh, hello," she replied, "what do you want? Is Charlotte okay?"

"She's fine," answered Charlie, "I just thought it best to let you know I'm going to court in a couple of days."

"So?" said Linda.

"Well," said Charlie, "should be okay at the first hearing, it'll probably be adjourned, but when I'm sentenced……"

"Have you been thieving again?"

"Nothing like that," replied Charlie, "bit of a misunderstanding with Julian Mason."

"Oh," said Linda, "what's it to do with me?"

"Well," answered Charlie, "worst case scenario: if I go to prison for a month or so, just need to be sure Charlotte will be okay."

"Course she will," snapped Linda, "I'll take care of her."

"Thanks," said Charlie.

"You'll never learn," said Linda, "will you?"

Charlie replaced the receiver. He never enjoyed his little chats with Linda.

A couple of days later, Charlie attended Dorking Magistrates' Court. Catherine, ever reliable, sat next to him in the waiting room.

"You'll be okay," said Catherine.

122

"I will be today," replied Charlie, "but if they want pre-sentence reports there's a good chance I'll go to prison when I come back."

Charlie yawned, then stretched, arms high and wide.

"You hit an old woman."

He turned and looked behind him. Two young lads sat a few yards away, laughing and joking. No old women. A quick check reassured him thatthere weren't any old ladies, anywhere in the room.

"What if she staggered out of the door?"

Charlie, stomach churning and heart racing, struggled to keep a lid on his anxiety. He turned to Catherine.

"Did you see me stretch out my arms?"

"Yes," she replied, "why?"

"Well," he said, "did anything strange happen?"

"Sorry?"

"I mean," said Charlie, "did I knock anyone or hit anyone?"

"No," replied Catherine.

"Are you sure?"

"Yes," answered Catherine, "the only people near us are the two lads sitting over there. And they haven't moved since we sat down."

The doubting disease gave a last shove.

"Would you swear to it?"

"I would," confirmed Catherine.

Charlie's anxiety lowered. Being sentenced in court…. no problem; living with constant doubt…….. demoralising.

A tall, slim gentleman, pin-striped suit, trendy glasses, grey hair and tanned complexion strode towards Charlie and Catherine. His left hand grasped a folder, bulging with paperwork.

"Hello," he said, "you must be Charlie."

"Yes," replied Charlie, "how do you know?"

"Process of elimination."

"Oh," said Charlie.

"I'm Mr. Neale," said the gent. "I hope you're aware that Mr. Gordon has retired."

"I had heard," replied Charlie.

"Well," continued Mr. Neale, "I'm here to represent you. I'm familiar with the case. Is that okay with you?"

"Fine ," answered Charlie.

Mr. Neale opened his folder and studied some paperwork.

"There's a free room along the corridor," he said, "we'd better have a chat."

"Okay," said Charlie, standing-up.

"Do you want me to come?" Catherine asked.

"No need," answered Mr. Neale, "this shan't take very long."

Charlie followed his new solicitor along the corridor.

"He puts me in mind of a professor," pondered Charlie.

They sat in a room, on either side of a wooden table.

"I'll come straight to the point," began Mr. Neale, "we'll ask for a fine but it's not very likely. They'll probably want reports."

"Okay," replied Charlie.

"I'll do my best," concluded Mr. Neale.

"That was bloody quick," thought Charlie, sitting next to Catherine in the waiting room, "he can't be paid an hourly rate. Must be the number of clients."

Within an hour, Charlie sat in the dock. Catherine watched from the viewing gallery. Mr. Neale delivered a short, but impressive, defence, but he didn't stand a chance. The presiding magistrate, sixty-five if a day, glared at Charlie. No conferring. No retiring for discussion. Immediate decision.

"We shall be requiring pre-sentence reports. This is a very serious matter. Bail will be extended. You may leave."

"Miserable fucker," thought Charlie, "I expected reports, but he didn't even think about it. Especially as Prof put in such a good performance."

Charlie met Catherine and Mr. Neale in the waiting room.

"Four weeks, Charlie," said Mr. Neale, "try and give a good account with the probation service. It'll make all the difference."

Days passed. Illnesses and assaults on elderly ladies caused much anxiety. Catherine, for most of the time, did a great reassurance job. Saturday morning, Charlotte at Linda's and Catherine doing a twelve hour shift.

Charlie studied the medical dictionary, anxiety rising.

"Neuralgia," he read, "pain in the face."

He flicked backwards through the pages.

"MS," he read, "the symptoms of MS………."

He read intently.

"A pain in the face can be a sign of MS," he panicked,

touching his cheek.

He read on.

"It's highly unlikely," he pondered, trying to relax, "that a slight ache in my cheek indicates MS."

"But what if it's the first sign? You could be crippled within a year."

An unsteady hand rubbed his thumping head.

"Look," he reasoned, "it's most likely neuralgia. Nothing more. Nothing less."

"But can't neuralgia be a sign of MS?"

"I think so," he mused, studying the text, "but rarely. Probably got a touch of neuralgia and that's that."

He went to his room and lay on the bed. His anxiety stayed high, adding to the pain in his forehead. An hour passed, Charlie felt slightly better.

"I'll take a couple of headache tablets," he decided, "and go for a short stroll. Won't be much fun without Tiger but it should help my head."

Charlie took two tablets, grabbed his knife, locked the door and left.

"Lucy and Hazel will be out 'til late," he remembered, "think they've gone visiting the old and frail."

He walked down the road.

"Bloody hell," he panicked, "hope I don't come across any old women."

He walked on, struggling with heightening anxiety.

"I won't go far," he decided. "It'd be much easier with Catherine to check for me."

A few more paces brought a loss of nerve, and Charlie turned and headed for home.

Chapter 9

As the door slammed shut, Charlie's anxiety levels started to decline. A cup of coffee and a roll-up….. that'd do the trick.

"Think I'll have another look at the medical book, read a bit more about MS. Knowledge is power."

There was a knock on the door.

"Who's that?" Charlie wondered.

He stood up and headed for the door. He pulled it open. Two men, mid-twenties, stood outside. Fairly ordinary, around six foot, short cropped hair, one medium build, the other a bit of a bloater. Both wore tee shirts, displaying a range of tattoos.

"Hello," said Charlie, "what can I do for you?"

Always best to be polite when you're not sure who you're talking to.

"Are you Charlie Lloyd?"

"Yeah," he answered.

The punch caught Charlie squarely on the nose. Blood dripped off his face as he staggered backwards. He blinked, trying to clear water from his eyes.

"Shit," he panicked, "what the fuck's happening?"

He felt dazed and completely disorientated, and struggled to stay on his feet.

Tubby and his mate were slow to move in for the kill.

"Can't exactly run for it," panicked Charlie, "what the fuck can I do?"

Tubby inched forwards, perhaps reluctant to finish, perhaps taking time to savour the moment. His friend stood a yard behind, seemingly waiting for a lead.

"Bloody hell," thought Charlie, adrenalin pumping through his system, "got to do something. They could fucking kill me."

A thought flashed into his mind. A saving grace? He hadn't done anything since his walk except make a coffee and roll a cigarette. He pulled the knife from his pocket and opened the blade. Arm outstretched, hand a little unsteady, he directed the blade towards Tubby.

"Stay there," snorted Charlie, ignoring the blood dripping from his nose.

"You wanker," jeered Tubby.

"We'll see," said Charlie, "just go."

"Yeah?"

"I would, "said Charlie.

A CRY FOR EVER

"Come on, Mark," said Tubby, "this cock ain't worth the bother."

Tubby and Mark walked through the open door. Tubby turned and took a last look at Charlie.

"You ain't heard the last of this."

Charlie stood, frozen to the spot, for almost a minute. Then, he shut the door and locked it. He checked every window, greatly relieved Tubby and co. seemed to have vanished. He went to the bathroom and held toilet tissue on his bleeding nose. Even with his head tilted, the blood kept coming.

"Fucking hell," he thought, "could be broken."

It took almost ten minutes to stem the flow.

"That's much better," pondered Charlie, "should be okay, now."

Just to be on the safe side, Charlie dabbed Vaseline up each nostril.

"Sure I'll be okay," he decided, "now, coffee and fag."

He sat at the kitchen table, drinking and smoking. Apart from a large cut on the bridge of his nose and slight swelling around the right eye, he was fine. He put his knife on the table without bothering to fold away the blade.

"What the fuck was that all about?"

He took a drag and sipped his coffee.

"It definitely wasn't a random attack," he pondered, "they asked my name then hit me."

Another drag, followed by a gulp.

"I'm absolutely certain I've never seen either of them before," he mused, "so someone must have sent them."

Another drag, then another.

"So, the question is," he pondered, "who sent them and how badly were they supposed to damage me?"

He crushed his roll-up in the ashtray.

"If they were supposed to put me in hospital," thought Charlie, "they didn't do a very good job. If, on the other hand, they just wanted to worry me, then they done okay."

He rolled another cigarette. A roll-up seemed to stimulate the brain.

"Now," he pondered, "who could have asked them to do me?"

A long drag, inhaling deeply.

"Would someone have got them to come here as a favour, or were they paid?"

He put his roll-up on the ashtray and paced the kitchen floor.

"Who doesn't like me?"

He turned and kept pacing.

"Hundreds of people," he thought, "bloody hundreds."

He sat at the table, relighting his roll-up.

"But who are the most likely candidates?"

He swigged his coffee.

"I suppose," he pondered, "Linda's not my biggest fan. She's a possibility."

Another swig and puff on roll-up.

"An obvious candidate would be Andrew, Lucy's dopey ex. He's got enough money to pay someone, and he's a bit of a dodgy fucker."

He paced the floor.

"And, of course, there's Clive Chew. He's got a lot of dodgy mates. He was with James Wiseman when I spoke to him. I wouldn't be surprised if either of them had something to do with it."

He slumped at the table.

"And last," he mused, "but by no means least, good old Julian. If he didn't take the money then he'd have a very good reason. And he could easily afford to pay someone."

He crushed his roll-up, stood up and plodded to his bedroom. Face still a little sore. He lay on his bed, staring at the ceiling. "What if you've hit somebody's grandma and they've come for revenge."

An intrusion was the last thing he wanted.

Charlie rolled on his stomach.

"Oh, fuck off," he muttered, " Every worry has been cleared. At this precise moment I don't have any."

Charlie headed for bed, long before Lucy and Hazel came home. He lay in the darkness, gently touching his aching face.

"Still ain't got a clue who's behind it," he murmured. "Let's hope, that'll be the end of the matter."

Names kept popping into his head, some possible, others ridiculous. He pretended to be asleep when Lucy and Hazel got back, but it was the early hours of the morning before he dozed. The slightest sound would trigger an immediate response: a return to his waking nightmare.

A CRY FOR EVER

Monday, mid-morning, Catherine parked outside Charlie's house. He opened the door.

"Hi," she said.

"Hello," replied Charlie.

"Blimey," she said, looking at his face, "what happened to you?"

"Walked into the door," replied Charlie.

"Really?"

"Well," said Charlie, "that's what I told Lucy and Hazel."

"So," said Catherine, "what really happened?"

"Two blokes knocked on the door," answered Charlie, "asked my name, then hit me."

"Serious?"

"Yeah," answered Charlie.

"Who were they? Why would they do that?"

"Haven't a clue," replied Charlie, "never seen them before."

"What did they say?"

"Not much," answered Charlie.

"Could they be friends of someone you've upset?"

"Quite possibly," replied Charlie.

"What about someone you've burgled in the past?"

"Hadn't given that much thought," answered Charlie, "but I suppose that could be possible."

"Who do you think?"

"Well," said Charlie, "there are a few obvious candidates."

"Such as?"

"Andrew, Lucy's dopey ex," said Charlie, "Clive Chew, Julian, or, I suppose, Linda could've asked someone. She's not my biggest fan."

"Bloody hell," said Catherine, "must be nice being so popular."

"I've been thinking about it all weekend," said Charlie, "nothing definite."

"Oh," replied Catherine.

"Tiger is watching Jungle Book," said Charlie. "how about a coffee?"

"Good idea," answered Catherine.

They sat at the table, drinking, smoking and chatting. Charlotte lay on the sofa, in the lounge, transfixed by Jungle Book……. yet again.

"Got probation reports on Thursday," said Charlie, "any

chance of a lift or have you got work?"

"I'm at work tomorrow and Wednesday," replied Catherine, "so Thursday will be fine."

"Great," said Charlie.

"Is Mr. Carson doing the report?"

"As far as I know," answered Charlie.

"What time?"

"We need to be there for two o'clock," answered Charlie.

After some toasted sandwiches, four cups of coffee and several roll-ups, Catherine suggested, "Shall we take Charlotte to the leisure centre?"

"Good idea," replied Charlie, "she's been watching videos all day. Crazy Tots or a swim would do her the world of good."

"Let's get going," said Catherine, draining the last of her coffee.

Wednesday lunchtime, and Charlotte was finishing her last piece of ham.

"Well done, Tiger," said Charlie, "at least you're eating has improved.

"Crisps," said Charlotte.

Charlie fetched a packet of salt and vinegar.

"Bit boring without Catherine," he commented.

"Yes," agreed Charlotte.

"She's doing a twelve hour shift," said Charlie, "bet she's knackered. Still, shell be here tomorrow."

Charlie stared out of the kitchen window. As he watched the trees blowing in the wind his vision, just for a second, lacked focus. He rubbed his eyes and blinked. Normal vision was restored.

"That was a bit odd," pondered Charlie, "my vision was a bit foggy."

He rolled a cigarette, diverting his thoughts. A failed attempt.

"Foggy! That could mean glaucoma! You could end up blind. Not much use to Charlotte."

His breathing became shallow and rapid. Mouth dry, heart thumping, head throbbing. A tingling sensation in fingers and toes.

"Bloody hell," he panicked, "could it be MS…….. again."

He fidgeted on his chair, desperate to keep control.

"Look," he tried to rationalise, "the blurred vision is just that, blurred vision, nothing else. You can check with Dr. King that you haven't got glaucoma. Even if you have, a few eye-drops and you'll be fine. Worst case scenario, an operation to relieve pressure in the eye."

He lit his roll-up. A major weapon in the struggle against anxiety.

"As for MS," he pondered, "pins and needles in your fingers and toes doesn't mean anything. Chances are, they are caused by the increase in your heartbeat. Hyperventilation syndrome."

He puffed furiously on his roll-up.

"Shall I have a quick peek in the medical book," he mused, "just to get my facts straight about glaucoma?"

Smoke filled the kitchen.

"Really shouldn't," he reasoned, "if I read about an illness, I'll get the symptoms."

He stood up, paced the kitchen, then sat down.

"Let's watch a video, Tiger," he said.

They settled down in front of the television.

"Hang on for a minute," said Charlie, "just got to look in my book."

"Okay," said Charlotte, glued to the screen.

Charlie, almost running, went to get the medical dictionary. He turned to glaucoma, hands more than a little unsteady.

"Symptoms," he read, "some fogginess of vision, aching pain in and above the eye…………."

He struggled with an overwhelming urge to panic.

"Look," he rationalised, "my vision was blurred for less than a second. I don't think I've ever had awful pain above or in my eye. I'm sure I haven't got glaucoma."

"What if you have? You could go blind?"

He shut the book.

"Fuck off," he muttered, "I'll check with Dr. King. Got an appointment next week. Even if I have got bloody glaucoma, I'll get it sorted. Now, I've got to concentrate on Tiger and make sure she's okay."

He sat for a few minutes, deep breaths controlling his anxiety.

"You okay, Tiger?" he asked, walking into the lounge, "enjoying the video?"

On Thursday, around twelve, Catherine parked outside Charlie's house. Charlie and Charlotte were drawing in the kitchen.

"Glad Catherine's not late," thought Charlie, "it wouldn't look good if I missed my probation appointment."

Catherine tapped on the door.

"Come in," shouted Charlie, "it's open."

Catherine walked into the kitchen and sat at the table.

"I'll make you a coffee," said Charlie, standing up.

"Thanks," replied Catherine.

"And I'll heat your spaghetti, Tiger."

Charlie and Catherine sat at the kitchen table, sipping coffee and puffing cigarettes. Charlotte sat on the sofa in the lounge, tucking into a bowl of spaghetti.

"Any idea who hit you?" Catherine asked.

"No," replied Charlie, "still ain't got a clue."

They both downed a second cup. Charlotte had finished her spaghetti and was watching Mr. Blobby on video. Catherine and Charlie had been gossiping for over an hour.

"Suppose we'd better make a move," said Charlie, "don't want to miss my turn."

"Okay," replied Catherine, standing up.

"Come on, Tiger," said Charlie, "we've got to go and see a man about a court case."

Charlie left Catherine and Charlotte in the waiting room, reading a book, and followed Mr. Carson to his room.

"So," began Mr. Carson, "as you know, I've got to write a report for the court before you're sentenced for the assault on Mr. Mason."

"Yes," said Charlie.

"Well," said Mr. Carson, "the offence was committed while you were on probation, so I think the court would be reluctant for another order."

"I see," said Charlie.

"As far as I'm aware, you're ineligible for community service," said Mr. Carson.

"That's right," answered Charlie.

"It is a serious offence," continued Mr. Carson.

"So," interrupted Charlie, "what can I expect?"

"Well," said Mr. Carson, "I haven't seen Dr. King's final report, but you should expect a short period in custody."

"How long?"

"I very much doubt it would be any longer than six months," answered Mr. Carson.

"Okay," said Charlie.

"Now," said Mr. Carson, "will your condition be manageable in custody?"

"Well," answered Charlie, "I'll be able to get my medication."

"I mean," explained Mr. Carson, "will custody cause a worsening of your condition?"

"No," answered Charlie, "it'll be okay."

"Right," said Mr. Carson, "the report will be ready when you go back to court."

"Okay," said Charlie.

"Your time with me will be finished after court," concluded Mr. Carson, "so I'd just like to wish you the very best for the future."

"Thank-you," replied Charlie, heading for the exit.

On the journey home, Catherine attempted conversation, but found Charlie very preoccupied.

"What did he say?"

"Not much," replied Charlie.

"Did he say what might happen in court?"

"Difficult to tell," answered Charlie, "but prison is definitely a possibility."

"Oh," said Catherine.

Charlotte, strapped in the backseat, gazed out the window.

"How about the Spice Girls, Charlotte," said Catherine, taking a tape from the glove compartment.

"Yes please," replied Charlotte.

Charlie stared at the road ahead trying to come to grips with his predicament.

"What a pain," he thought, "if I get six months, then I'll have to serve at least three. Tiger will be living at Linda's all that time. When I get out, she might want to stay with Linda."

He rolled a cigarette.

"Fuck," he thought, "I've really made a mess of things. I'm not much good to Tiger if I'm sitting in prison."

The car parked outside Charlie's house.

"Home, sweet home," said Catherine, "time for a coffee."

Saturday afternoon. No Catherine and no Charlotte. Charlie watched rugby on the television. There was a sharp knock on the door.

"Bloody hell," panicked Charlie, recalling his unwanted visitors, "I'm not expecting anyone."

He rushed to his room, pocketed his knife, then, cautiously, opened the door. Hand in pocket, he felt reassured by the feel of the knife.

"Hello," said Edward, "how are things?"

"Hi," replied Charlie, anxiety ebbing away, "really good to see you."

They chatted, drank coffee and smoked roll-ups.

"Got court on the twenty-eighth," said Charlie.

"Two weeks," said Edward, "what day is the twenty-eighth?"

"It's a Tuesday," answered Charlie.

"Haven't got any plans," said Edward, "I'll come and give you some support."

"Really?"

"Yeah," answered Edward, "you'll make a right mess of things if I'm not with you."

"Okay," said Charlie, "that'd be really good."

"What do you reckon you'll get? Fine?"

"Probably get put away," answered Charlie.

"You're joking," said Edward, "he only lost a few teeth and got a little bump behind his ear."

"I know," replied Charlie, "but when I saw the probation officer he said a short custodial sentence."

"Fuck that," said Edward. "I still think you might be okay."

"Time will tell," replied Charlie.

A few more coffees and lots of cigarettes.

"Better get going," said Edward, "got a date this evening."

"Okay," replied Charlie.

"I'll see you in court," said Edward.

"Okay," repeated Charlie, "have a good night."

"I intend to," answered Edward.

Sunday lunchtime, and Charlie was home alone. Lucy was meeting a mystery man and Hazel was visiting relatives. Charlie felt anxious....... unexplained anxiety. He paced the kitchen.

"Got to get a grip," he urged, "nothing to worry about. No old women and no terminal illnesses."

He slumped at the table and rolled a cigarette. Gradually, his rapid breathing slowed and his heartbeat returned to normal. He dragged on his roll-up. A slight pounding in his head. He rubbed his forehead. Definitely, a throbbing headache.

"That's nasty. Probably got a brain tumour."

Heartbeat increased. Breathing quickened, becoming shallow.

A CRY FOR EVER

"Look," he urged, "think logically. Headaches are very common. Probably one of the most common complaints. It's extremely rare for a headache to indicate a serious problem."

Several quick drags on the roll-up.

"My head does hurt," he reasoned, "but it's probably brought on by stress."

He crushed his roll-up in the ashtray, fighting the urge to reach for the medical dictionary.

"Right," he thought, "I'll take a couple of painkillers and have a lie down. No need to look up brain tumour, as it'll give me lots more to worry about. If I'm still not happy, I can ask Dr. King at my next appointment."

Charlie downed the tablets with a glass of water and headed for the bedroom.

Monday morning, beginning of the week, Charlie pushed the swing as Charlotte giggled and kept forgetting to hold on. Forty minutes and Charlie's arms had started to ache.

"Better go home in a minute," said Charlie, "'cause Catherine is coming round today."

"Yes," giggled Charlotte.

Back home, coffee for Charlie. A cheese sandwich and a glass of blackcurrant juice for Charlotte. It wasn't long before a car parked outside the house.

"Catherine's here," said Charlie, opening the door.

"Hi," said Catherine.

A quick coffee and a couple of cigarettes.

"Shall we take Charlotte to Brocketts Farm?"

"Good idea," answered Charlie, "she'll love it."

A lovely afternoon out ended just before five o'clock. Back at the kitchen table, they had coffee, cigarettes, blackcurrant juice and shepherd's pie. Charlotte, exhausted, managed an hour's television before surrendering to the inevitable sleep.

"Have you got an appointment with Dr. King tomorrow?"

"Yeah," replied Charlie, "he'll be doing a report for court."

"What time?"

"Seeing him at four o'clock," answered Charlie.

"I can take you," said Catherine, "if it's okay, I'll stay tonight. I'm not working 'til Friday."

"Great," replied Charlie.

"Where are Lucy and Hazel?"

"Lucy has got a mystery boyfriend," replied Charlie, "and Hazel has gone for a meal with a friend."

Even caffeine stimulation failed to keep Catherine and Charlie awake past ten thirty. A day on the farm......... they just couldn't handle the pace.

The following morning, an early start.....Charlotte rarely slept past seven. A quiet day, colouring and watching videos.

"It's after three," said Charlie, downing his coffee, "better make a move."

"Okay," replied Catherine, "can't keep Dr. King waiting."

Charlie sat opposite Dr. King, waiting for the psychiatrist to speak..

"So," said Dr. King, "how have you been?"

"Okay," said Charlie, "still keep worrying about different illnesses."

"How long does each worry last?"

"Well," answered Charlie, "'til they're cleared by the passing of time, reassurance or replaced by another worry."

"So," said Dr. King, "it's affecting daily living?"

"Yeah," replied Charlie, "always got something on my mind."

"What's been bothering you recently?"

"I've been worried about glaucoma and a brain tumour," answered Charlie.

"What's made you think that?"

"I had blurred vision," replied Charlie, "and I've been getting quite a few headaches."

"Was the blurred vision temporary?"

"Just for a few seconds," answered Charlie.

"Not glaucoma," said Dr. King, "probably nothing."

"Can you be sure?"

"Any loss of vision? Throbbing behind your eyes?"

"No," answered Charlie.

"It really is highly unlikely," soothed Dr. King.

"You think?"

"Well," said Dr. King, "I wouldn't waste my life worrying about something that'll probably never happen."

"Yeah, suppose," answered Charlie.

"What about the headaches?"

"Well," answered Charlie, "I've been getting loads of them."

"So," said Dr. King, "why would they be caused by a tumour?"

"Well," replied Charlie, "lots of headaches can indicate a

serious problem."

"True," said Dr. King, "these types of headache are usually a certain type, at certain times of the day. In your case, the obvious cause would be stress."

"You reckon?"

"Well," replied Dr. King, "if you spend all day worrying about various conditions, then I'm not in the least bit surprised you suffer with headaches. I'd be more surprised if you didn't."

"Oh," said Charlie.

Dr. King took a sip of water from a glass on his desk.

"I've been asked to write a court report for you," he said.

"Yeah," replied Charlie, "I know."

"Actual bodily harm?"

"That's right," answered Charlie.

"Did your condition have any bearing on your offence?"

"No," replied Charlie, "it didn't."

"Will prison worsen your problems?"

"No," answered Charlie, "shouldn't do."

"Okay," said Dr. King, "I'll write a report and we'll see what happens."

"Right," replied Charlie.

"Is the case next week?"

"Yeah," replied Charlie.

"I'll see you after the case," said Dr. King, smiling, "or when sentence has been served."

"Yeah," answered Charlie.

"Make a note of any illnesses," concluded Dr. King, "and we'll discuss them next time."

Days passed; each seemed shorter than the previous one. It was Saturday lunchtime, a bright, clear day, but Charlie's mood darkened his outlook.

"Court on Tuesday," he pondered, flicking through the television channels, "what if I get six months and lose contact with Tiger?"

A rugby match played to a packed house on channel one.

"Can't do much about it now," he pondered.

A conversion was successful.

"Hope Catherine is having a good shift at work."

A forward was carried off the pitch holding his head.

"Wonder what Tiger is doing at Linda's," he pondered.

The phone rang, interrupting a fluent move near the posts.

"Hi," said Debbie, "how are you?"

"Oh, not too bad," replied Charlie, "how's the job at the bakery?"

"Oh," answered Debbie, "got the sack."

"Why?"

"Kept giving people the wrong change," replied Debbie.

"Oh," said Charlie, "never mind."

"What's been happening with you?"

"Got court on Tuesday," answered Charlie, "getting sentenced for bopping Julian."

"What do you reckon will happen?"

"Not sure," answered Charlie, "worst case scenario - six months."

"Oh," said Debbie, "well, I haven't any plans for Tuesday, so I'll come with you."

"Okay," said Charlie, "if you want."

"Can I have a lift with you and Catherine?"

"Should be fine," replied Charlie, "I'll check with her and let you know."

"Great," said Debbie.

Chapter 10

Tuesday, as usual, followed Monday. Charlie and Catherine rolled out of bed before seven. Plenty of time for caffeine and nicotine before the court case. Charlotte slept soundly. Worrying about a silly court case wasn't on the menu.

"Let's have a coffee and a fag before we wake Tiger," said Charlie, heading for the kitchen.

"Good idea," replied Catherine.

Charlie poured two steaming cups.

"What time we got to be there?"

"I've got to answer bail at nine o'clock," answered Charlie.

"What time shall we leave?"

"Well," replied Charlie, "got to drop Tiger at Linda's and collect Debbie. Better leave around eight."

"Okay," said Catherine.

Charlie drained his second cup of coffee.

"Just go and get sorted," he said, heading to the bathroom, "then we'll wake Tiger."

He washed, cleaned his teeth, then dressed. Clean sweatshirt and dungarees.

"Cath," he called, finished in the bathroom."

He gently shook Charlotte.

"Tiger," he whispered, "wake up."

Charlotte stirred, yawned, then climbed from her bed.

"Morning, Tiger," said Charlie, "what can I get you for breakfast?"

Hazel and Lucy, ten minutes apart, clambered out of bed, had a cup of tea and a slice of toast, and left for work.

Charlotte finished a second bowl of cornflakes. She dressed and sat in the lounge enthralled by children's television.

Fifteen minutes to eight and Catherine emerged ready for the day ahead.

"Time for one last coffee before we go," said Charlie.

"Why not?"

They dropped Charlotte at Linda's.

"Bye, Tiger," said Charlie, "have a lovely time with Mummy."

"Bye," said Charlotte.

"Won't be long," said Charlie, "and I'll be round to get you."

"Yes," said Charlotte.

"Be good," said Charlie, turning away.

STEPHEN DRAKE

As he climbed into the car, he felt like he had swallowed a gobstopper.

"Get a grip," he scolded himself, "nobody's died. Even if the worst happens, you'll be back in three months."

He slumped into the passenger seat and fastened his seatbelt.

"Right," he said, "let's go and get Debbie."

Debbie was ready, smartly presented, fag hanging out her mouth.

"You okay, Charlie?"

"Yeah," replied Charlie, "bit nervous."

They drove along the roads, relieved not to encounter heavy traffic.

"Will anyone else be coming?" Debbie asked.

"Ed said he'd try and turn up," answered Charlie.

"Reckon he will?"

"I hope so," answered Charlie, "be nice if he did."

They parked behind a white van about twenty yards from the court building.

"Here we go," said Charlie.

"You'll be fine," replied Catherine.

They headed towards the entrance. Five yards from the door, stooped and grey, an old lady fumbled in her handbag.

"Oh shit," thought Charlie, considering his options.

He grasped his dungaree straps. Both hands were accounted for - check! He took a hasty diversion, putting at least three yards between himself and the lady. Passing caused an increase in anxiety but not a loss of control. As he opened the glass door, he looked back. The old lady, completely unharmed and blissfully unaware of any problem, rummaged deeper in her bag.

"She's fine," thought Charlie, "no worries."

Charlie, Catherine and Debbie found three empty seats towards the front of the waiting room. Other defendants scattered the room, most appearing uncomfortable in smart attire. A small stall, in the corner, sold coffee, tea, juice and biscuits.

"Edward's not here," said Debbie.

"Hopefully he'll turn up later," replied Charlie.

It wasn't long before a list of defendants were called to court one to surrender to bail.

"You must stay in the waiting room," announced the

magistrate, "until you are called for your case to be heard. You may not leave the building."

Charlie went to join Catherine and Debbie in the waiting room. He was delighted to see Edward, sitting next to Debbie, sipping a coffee and munching a biscuit.

"Hello mate," said Edward.

"Hi," said Charlie.

"How you feeling?"

"Bit nervous," replied Charlie. "I really don't want to go to prison. Usually, I couldn't care what happens."

"Sure you'll be fine," said Edward, "don't think you'll get put away for a couple of punches."

Charlie stood up.

"Just going for a piss," he said.

Charlie returned to his seat, slumped next to Catherine and waited.

"When I was waiting to take French oral for common entrance," he pondered, "I was shitting myself. Just trying to decide if this is worse."

The loudspeaker made an almost inaudible sound.

"Barker. Court one."

A young lad, no older than twenty, scruffy haircut but smart clothes, stood up and walked into court one.

"Well," said Edward, "things have started. Soon be over."

"Need a slash," said Charlie, climbing to his feet.

Charlie walked back into the waiting room and sat down.

Mr. Neale approached the group.

"Where the fuck did he appear from?" thought Charlie, only noticing his solicitor when he was within touching distance.

"Hello," said Mr. Neale.

"Hi," said Charlie.

"There's a free room down the corridor," stated Mr. Neale, "we'd better take this opportunity to have a chat."

"Okay," replied Charlie, following his solicitor to the consulting room.

They sat in the room, either side of a large wooden table.

"Right," began Mr. Neale, clearing his throat, "I have the reports so we'll be able to proceed."

"That's good," said Charlie.

"There's a question I feel I have to ask," said Mr. Neale.

"Yeah," replied Charlie.

"Would you be prepared to pay compensation to Mr. Mason for the injuries he sustained?"

"Well............" Charlie hesitated.

"It would count very strongly in your favour," encouraged Mr. Neale.

Charlie squirmed uncomfortably on his chair.

"Shit," he pondered, "now what do I do? If I agree to pay, it'll look like I'm admitting I've made a mistake. Maybe Julian didn't take the money. It's quite possible somebody else was nicking. If I pay him, everything will have been for nothing. I'll look a right mug."

"Mr. Lloyd......."

"Sorry," replied Charlie, "I was just thinking about what you said."

"And?"

"Well," said Charlie, "I really don't think paying compensation would be fair on me."

"Why?"

"He's already had the money," said Charlie, trying to convince himself.

"It wouldn't be more than eighty pounds," pushed Mr. Neale.

"No, I can't," said Charlie.

"Well," said Mr. Neale, "it's going to be difficult keeping you out of custody."

"Oh," stammered Charlie.

"I will do my best," concluded Mr. Neale, "but you appreciate my hands are tied."

The solicitor stood up, gathered his papers and opened the door.

"Fuck," thought Charlie, standing up, "hope I'm doing the right thing. Eighty quid and no prison. No chance of losing Tiger. But, I'll look a cock and all this would've been for nothing. Someone's been nicking Tiger's money and getting away with it."

Charlie followed his solicitor back to the waiting room. A lady stood by the door, tears streaming down her face. Charlie sat between Debbie and Edward.

"What's wrong with her?"

"Think her son has just been sent to prison," answered Edward.

"What for?"

"I heard her talking earlier; he'd been driving on a ban,"

replied Edward.

"Shit," said Charlie, "is that all?"

"Yeah," replied Edward, "but I think he was caught twice."

"What court was he in?"

"One," answered Edward, "same as you."

"Fuck," muttered Charlie.

The loudspeaker disturbed Charlie's darkening mood.

"West. Court Two."

"Just going for a leak," announced Charlie, struggling to his feet.

"Wow," said Catherine, smiling, "you are nervous."

Charlie hadn't been back in his seat for five minutes when the loudspeaker crackled an announcement.

"Lloyd. Court one."

"Fuck," murmured Charlie.

"Good luck, mate," said Edward.

"Best of luck, Charlie," said Catherine, with a comforting pat on his shoulder.

"Hope it's okay," said Debbie, wiping her eyes.

Bloody hell," thought Charlie, looking at Debbie, "she's in tears. Oh well, at least she cares."

Charlie opened the door, walked anxiously into the courtroom and took position in the dock. Edward, Catherine and Debbie settled in the public gallery. The three magistrates watched intently. Charlie glanced at the trio, trying to feel a vibe. Two middle-aged women either side of an elderly gent.

"The women look okay," pondered Charlie, "quite sexy, actually."

He looked at the gent, presiding magistrate for the case. Fairly old, nearing retirement, decent head of dark hair, probably dyed, old-fashioned glasses perched on a long, pointed nose. Thin lips and large forehead suggested a fearsome disciplinarian.

"Blimey," thought Charlie, "don't like the look of him. Reminds me of an old headmaster of mine who caned anything that moved. He scared the shit out of me."

The court usher took a sheet from the clerk and handed it to the magistrates. The clerk looked more suited to a porn film. He was a handsome lad with blonde hair, fresh features and body of an athlete. The usher looked as if she lived in a retirement home. She was an old woman, past retirement, with grey hair, hearing aid and dodgy leg.

"Oh, fuck," thought Charlie, gripping his dungaree straps, "that's all I need."

"Could you stand properly, please," said Headmaster, "with your hands down."

"Looks can be deceptive," thought Charlie, lowering his arms, "but, in this case........"

"Sit down please, Mr. Lloyd," stated Headmaster, "we are ready to proceed."

Charlie sat in the dock, eyes front. The prosecuting solicitor, a tall man, muscular build complete with flattened nose, adjusted some papers.

"Looks like a boxer," pondered Charlie, "wouldn't fancy meeting him down a dark alley."

Rocky took to his feet and cleared his throat. Round one.

"A serious assault...... blah.... ...blah............. premeditated......... blah........lured into an ambush.............blah..........concealed identity..............blah...............runaway with complete disregard for victim....................."

"Bloody hell," thought Charlie, "he's making me sound so callous. Six months...... get ready. Might even be referred to Crown Court for sentence."

Rocky, opponent on the ropes, threw a vicious hook.

"Refused to pay compensation, demonstrating a complete lack of remorse."

Charlie shifted uneasily in the dock. Headmaster stared intently at Rocky, absorbing every word.

"So," concluded Rocky, "I would urge the court to appreciate the serious nature of this offence.

Rocky sat down, satisfied with an impressive performance.

"Come on, Mr. Neale," muttered Charlie, "time to earn your extortionate wages."

Mr. Neale stood up, took a sip of water and glanced at his papers.

"Mr. Lloyd admitted the offence early in the case....... blah....blah..... not at the serious end of the scale........blah.....blah..................Mr. Lloyd has been a very conscientious father........blah.....blah....... alternatives to a prison sentence........."

"Well," mused Charlie, "he certainly tried. Question is, has he done enough?"

Charlie glanced at the public gallery. Catherine sat upright, staring at the bench. Debbie slumped forward, chewing her nails. A thumbs-up from Edward.

Mr. Neale and Rocky, both seated, waited for Headmaster to dictate proceedings. Finally, he broke the silence.

"Am I to understand that Mr. Lloyd was asked to pay compensation but declined?"

"Er..... well......yes," stammered Mr. Neale, "Mr. Lloyd viewed his actions as summary justice, and consequently declined the offer to pay compensation."

"Shit," thought Charlie, watching his solicitor, "reckon I've really fucked-up. I could have got the wrong person, and not paying compensation could cost me. Too fucking stubborn."

"Thank-you, Mr. Neale," said Headmaster.

Mr. Neale sat down. He'd fought a good battle with very limited weapons.

"We shall retire to consider our verdict," announced Headmaster.

The magistrates filed out the court, giving everyone temporary relaxation.

Mr. Neale walked over to the dock.

"Okay?"

"Yeah," replied Charlie, "how do you think it went?"

"Not too bad," answered Mr. Neale, "all we can do is wait."

"Yeah," said Charlie.

"I think," said Mr. Neale, "if you get longer than three months we should lodge an appeal."

"Okay," said Charlie, "how long do you reckon they'll be?"

"How long is a piece of string?"

Mr. Neale walked over to the prosecution, leaving Charlie to consider his fate. He watched his solicitor and Rocky laughing and joking.

It's all a big game to them," he thought, "bit friendly for two people on opposite sides. Still, it's money in the bank, whatever happens."

Charlie glanced towards the public gallery trying to establish eye contact. Bit of reassurance wouldn't go amiss. The trio averted his gaze. Why say anything if you haven't anything positive to say! Charlie conceded defeat and focused on the floor.

"I really need a piss," he thought, "hope they hurry up."

He crossed his legs and waited. And waited. Deliberations had already lasted over an hour.

"Hope Tiger's okay," pondered Charlie, "really hope I get to see her later."

The usher walked past the dock. Instinctively, Charlie grabbed his dungaree straps. He watched her carefully as she conferred with the clerk.

"She's fine," he muttered, releasing his grip, "no worries."

He rubbed his forehead; a slight ache could signify worse to follow.

"Bollocks," he thought, "I really don't need a headache at this precise moment. 'Suppose it must be all the bloody stress."

He stared at the floor and waited. And waited. Deliberations had taken nearly three hours. Charlie's bladder would testify to that.

"Better not leave the dock for a piss," decided Charlie, "and there's nobody to ask. Hope I don't wet myself. I'll be a laughing stock. If I go to prison a village will be without its idiot."

He glanced at the public gallery. Edward stared at the dock.

"You'll be okay," he mouthed, "don't think they'll send you away."

"Not sure," mouthed Charlie, shrugging his shoulders, "never know."

The longer the wait, the higher the anxiety. Not ideal when you're desperate for a slash.

The bell tolled, signalling a decision had been made. The magistrates filed back into the court room. Charlie gazed at Headmaster, trying to gauge an indication of the result of their deliberations.

"He doesn't look happy," thought Charlie, "still, he hasn't smiled all day."

Headmaster licked his lips, then cleared his throat.

"Stand up, please, Mr. Lloyd."

Charlie took to his feet. A little unsteady, nagging headache and bladder full to capacity.

"Just get on with it," urged Charlie, under his breath, "put me out my misery."

Charlie noticed a policeman lurking, at the door, behind the dock. As he would leave the court room through that door, it suggested that going home was not on the agenda.

"Bugger," panicked Charlie, "not a good sign. Usually, if they call for a jailer, you're going to prison."

He took a quick look at the constable, big bloke, mid twenties, short dark hair and an eye patch.

"Somebody didn't fancy a trip to jail," pondered Charlie, staring at the eye patch, "wonder what happened?"

He focused his attention on the bench. Wouldn't be wise to annoy Headmaster.

"That's strange," thought Charlie, eyes flicking between magistrates, "wonder what's happen to John."

"We have listened carefully," stated Headmaster, "to the prosecution's case, and taken into consideration what has been said by the defence. We have decided not to make a compensation order for the offence. However, we are of the opinion, this is a serious, pre-meditated assault aggravated by a failure to comply with community sentences. We sentence you to twenty-eight days in prison."

The policeman stood next to Charlie, hand resting on his shoulder.

"Come with me," said the constable, leading Charlie from the dock.

Before the door slammed shut, Charlie took a last look at the public gallery. Edward sat forward, head resting on hands, looking bemused. Catherine stood slowly, wondering what to do. Debbie, tears streaming down her face, searched her bag for a tissue.

"Fucking hell," thought Charlie, looking at Debbie, "it's only a month. I'm not complaining, could have been much worse."

Charlie followed the policeman to the cell-block. The first cell was occupied. Young lad, late teens, short and skinny, messy haircut.

"Looks like he's been crying," thought Charlie, noticing his swollen eyes and red face.

The second cell was also taken. Another young lad, no more than twenty. Tall, athletic build, shaved head and tattoos etched on every exposed area.

Charlie was shown to cell three. At least he didn't have to share. He turned to the constable before the door was locked.

"What happened to John, the jailer who used to work here?"

"He hasn't worked for nearly a year," replied the officer, "has a few health problems."

"Oh," said Charlie, "if you speak to him, please offer him my best wishes. He'll remember me......... Charlie Lloyd."

"Okay," replied the officer.

"What happened to your eye? Prisoner with the hump?"

"No," answered the policeman, "a colleague drank too much at a birthday bash."

"Oh dear," said Charlie.

The officer slammed the door. Charlie sat on the bench. Prison van shouldn't be long.

"I'm in the cell next door to you."

"Yeah," answered Charlie.

"Have you been sent down today?"

"Yeah," said Charlie, "only got a month."

"I'm on remand. Been in Reading Prison for last five months."

"Reading?"

"Yeah, I'm only nineteen. They've got a Y.P. wing up there."

"When I was a Y.P.," replied Charlie, "they sent you to Lewes."

"Not now, mate. Everyone under twenty-one goes to Reading."

"Didn't know that," answered Charlie, "what's your name?"

"Terry."

"I'm Charlie."

Charlie made a skinny roll-up.

"What you done? How long you expecting?"

"Street robbery," answered Terry, "got hold of this lad, took his jacket, wallet, Walkman, jewellery, and slapped him a few times."

"Oh."

"Solicitor reckons," continued Terry, "could get five years."

"Oh," said Charlie, "and what about geezer in next cell?"

"He got done for driving on a ban," answered Terry, "first time in prison. Think he's in a bit of a state."

"Oh."

The cell opened. The policeman stood at the door.

"Got a light, governor?" Charlie said, holding his roll-up.

"Yeah," replied the officer, handing Charlie a lighter.

Charlie lit his roll-up and returned the lighter.

"Thanks," he said.

"You'll be leaving soon," said the officer, "you're the only one going to Highdown, so a couple of coppers will take you there."

"Okay," answered Charlie.

Charlie sat in the back of the police car, squeezed between two overweight constables.

"How long you got?"

"Only a month," replied Charlie.

"That'll fly by."

"Hope so," said Charlie.

He had to go through twenty-five minutes of forced conversation.

"Here we are."

"I remember it," replied Charlie, gazing at the outer walls.

"Let's get you inside."

"Twenty-eight days," pondered Charlie, "only serve fourteen. Lots can go wrong in a fortnight!"

Chapter 11

An hour in a cage. A radio blared down the corridor. Processed, strip-searched, left in another cage, slightly larger. Allocated kit. Visit to the doctor.

"Are you addicted to any drugs?"

"No," replied Charlie.

"Are you suicidal?"

"No," replied Charlie.

"Have you been convicted?"

"Yes."

"What for?"

"Actual bodily harm."

"Was it a member of your family?"

"No."

"How long is your sentence?"

"Month."

"Any medication?"

"Yeah," answered Charlie, "have three sulpiride tablets daily. Two hundred mg."

"I'll inform the wing," concluded the doctor.

Another cage, radio still blaring along the corridor. Charlie was joined by three other inmates. The first two prisoners had been sentenced for the same crime. Two black lads, early twenties, tall, athletically built.

"Bastard judge," cursed one, "twelve years."

"Bit of a shock," replied his co-defendant, "stabbing the shop manager...... attempted murder! It was only a flesh wound."

"Trouble is...... if you go tooled-up to do a bit of thieving...... you're in shit."

The third inmate, white, filthy clothes, was much older than his fellow convicts.

"What a state," pondered Charlie, "looks like he ain't washed for weeks. Must be an alcoholic, living rough. Probably got done for a bit of petty thieving and couldn't give an address."

A warden opened the cage.

"Right lads," he said, "let's go."

The four prisoners followed the officer along a maze of corridors. Steel bars separated them from the perfectly tended gardens. Even above their heads, more bars.

"It'd be almost impossible to escape," pondered Charlie, quickening his step, "how the fuck do these people do it?"

They turned a corner, passed the library, shelves of literature enclosed in a ring of steel, and followed a sign to house-block three.

"Four on," shouted their escort.

Two wardens appeared from the office, central on the unit. Both white, burly, one with big ears and the other with massive lips.

"Follow me," said Lips to Charlie, handing him a card, "cell twenty-one, landing three."

"Okay, guv," replied Charlie.

Charlie, bed-pack in hand, followed Lips up the stairs to landing three. Lips opened cell twenty-one, displayed Charlie's card outside, and locked him inside. Usual set-up, two beds, one on either side of the cell, with a small walkway between. At the far end of the cell was a small barred window. Under the window was a wooden table with two chairs. To the left of the door, separated by a flimsy partition, was a toilet. As Charlie stood by the door, his cell-mate stood up. A black lad, early twenties, around six foot, slim build but muscular. Shaved head.

"Not big," thought Charlie, "but it's all muscle. No fat on him. Could be a lightweight boxer."

The lad stared at Charlie, not blinking and not speaking.

"Obviously not a great conversationalist," decided Charlie, a little uneasy.

The lad rubbed his chin, checking his designer stubble. Still no introduction.

"Hello, mate," began Charlie, pointing at the bed on the left, "can I take this one?"

"Sure," replied his cell-mate.

Charlie laid his kit on the bed.

"I'm Charlie," he said.

"Owen," replied his cell-mate.

"How long you got?"

"I'm on remand," answered Owen, "been here for three weeks."

"What you expecting?"

"Seven years," replied Owen, "solicitor reckons could get ten years but if I'm lucky might only get five."

"Blimey," said Charlie, "what you done?"

"Got nicked at the airport trying to smuggle drugs."

"Oh," said Charlie.

"What about you?"

"Got a month," answered Charlie, "for fighting."

"Been in before?"

"Few times," replied Charlie, "for nicking."

Charlie made his bed, sat down and rolled a cigarette, thankful the officer in reception had turned a blind eye and allowed him to keep his open tobacco.

"Do you want a roll-up?"

"Yeah," replied Owen, "thanks."

Owen rolled a skinny cigarette and inhaled deeply. Charlie watched as smoke rings filled the cell.

"Have you been in before?"

"No," answered Owen, "had community service, bit of probation, loads of fines, but never prison."

Midnight came and went. Charlie and Owen smoked roll-ups and swapped stories. A general babble could be heard through the barred window. Inmates don't travel far, so early nights aren't a priority.

"Woof, woof, woof, woof."

"What the fuck's that?"

"Oh," replied Owen, "this happens every night. There's some loon on the other unit. Thinks he's a dog. Barks every night."

"How long?"

"Carries on for about an hour," answered Owen.

"Fucking hell," said Charlie.

"Should be in hospital," said Owen.

"Do you know anything about him?"

"Bit his father's face and throat," replied Owen, "nearly killed him. Best to keep out of his way."

"Woof, woof."

"You'll get used to it," said Owen.

It was almost four o'clock before Charlie fell asleep. Angry voices and laughter filled the night air for a long time afterwards. Charlie spent the night with Catherine and Charlotte on a sunny day at the park. Sweet dreams!

First morning, waking in prison, never easy to adjust.

"Breakfast, lads," said Lips, unlocking the door, "ten

minutes."

Charlie struggled from his pit, pulled on his dungarees, grabbed his plastics and left the cell. Owen buried his head under the covers. Charlie joined the queue for the nurse, collected his medication and waited at the barred gate for breakfast. After a bowl of tasteless porridge and cup of flavourless tea, Charlie was banged up for the morning. Owen still lay in his bed, snoring softly.

"Best way," thought Charlie, glancing at his cell-mate, "longer you're asleep, less time you serve."

Owen stirred around ten o'clock. He sat up in bed and rubbed his eyes. Rolled a cigarette and set himself for the boredom ahead.

"Morning, mate," said Charlie.

"Did you go to breakfast?"

"Yeah," answered Charlie, "porridge."

"Surprise, surprise," said Owen.

"You fucking cock!"

Charlie, heart racing and stomach churning, ground his teeth and held a clenched fist over his mouth.

"Shit," he panicked, "where the fuck did that come from?"

He watched intently as Owen puffed his second roll-up that morning. No reaction. Perfectly relaxed. Not the behaviour of someone suffering verbal abuse.

"He's fine," reasoned Charlie, "it was only a bloody thought."

"Got a good book about true crimes," said Owen, "do you want to read it?"

"Yeah," replied Charlie, "I'll have a look."

He took the book from his cell-mate.

"No worries," thought Charlie, "no fucking worries."

"Lunch, lads," said Lips, pushing open the door, "serving in about an hour.

"Reckon I'll get a shower," said Charlie to Owen, "feeling a bit grotty."

Charlie, holding his towel and soap, headed along the landing to the shower block. Nobody was about.

"Good," thought Charlie, "much prefer having a shower in peace."

He stood under the shower, enjoying the sensation of the warm water. All good things must come to an end. The door opened and he had company. A skinny prisoner, messy, shoulder-length hair and haggard features. Wearing shorts.

He displayed several homemade tattoos.

"Probably about thirty," decided Charlie, "but he's such a state, looks over fifty."

He walked to the far shower, bloated belly exaggerated by such a puny body.

"Not exactly a hunk," thought Charlie, "makes me look handsome."

Could things get worse? Yes! The prisoner opened his mouth.

"Bloody hell," thought Charlie, trying not to stare, "he's only got about three teeth in his whole mouth. And they look as rotten as fuck."

Every two or three seconds the prisoner glanced nervously at the door.

"He's worried about something," thought Charlie, "don't reckon I'll talk to him. Sense he's in trouble."

The door opened. A white inmate, dressed in blue jeans and striped shirt, walked in. A huge man, bald head, scarred face and covered in tattoos.

"Blimey," thought Charlie, "he's fucking massive. At least seventeen stone of muscle. No neck. Looks like someone has sliced his cheek. What about the tattoos...... hands, face, neck...... covered. He's even got a little dolphin on the side of his head."

The prisoner closed the door. He obviously didn't want to be disturbed.

"Fucking hell," thought Charlie, "he's not here for a shower. Hasn't even got a towel."

The inmate stared at Toothless, who struggled into his shorts.

"Got my burn?"

"I'll get it," whimpered Toothless, "just give me a week."

"No fucking chance!"

"Bloody hell," thought Charlie, adrenalin pumping, "he's in major strife."

Toothless looked terrified, visibly shaking, as the prisoner strode towards him. The first punch, hand like a slab of concrete, covered his face. His head jerked violently, he staggered backwards, collapsed against the wall and slid to the floor. His blood was diluted by the running shower.

"Fucking hell," thought Charlie, heart pounding, "he'll be lucky to have any teeth after this."

A CRY FOR EVER

The prisoner advanced on the pitiful wreck. It was like a drunken husband beating his wife after twelve pints down the local. Hand filled face and head crashed into shower floor.

"Not sure what to do," thought Charlie, fighting any outward displays of panic, "if I leave the shower block, it'll look like I'm shitting it. Worse still, he might think I'm a grass. Don't want to get involved…. ain't got nothing to do with me."

The beating finished. The prisoner, pleased with his work, left the showers. Toothless lay on the floor, face covered in blood, groaning softly.

"Least he ain't dead," thought Charlie, "best just to fuck off. Someone will find him in a minute."

Charlie dried himself, dressed quickly and left the showers.

He joined the queue waiting for the culinary delights on offer.

That afternoon, having survived pie and runny mash, Charlie and Owen chatted during bang-up.

Someone got a bit of a beating in the showers," said Charlie.

"Oh."

"Skinny geezer, bit of a mess, hardly any teeth….."

"Oh," said Owen, "they call him Gums. What happened?"

"Well," said Charlie, "he was having a shower and another bloke came in and beat the hell out of him."

"Who?"

"He was a big bloke, built like a shit-house, no neck, tattoos everywhere, bald head….."

"That's Tank," interrupted Owen, "a mean fucker."

"What was it over?"

"A game of pool," answered Owen.

"How come?"

"They had a bet," said Owen, "half an ounce. Tank won."

"And Gums didn't pay?"

"Well," said Owen, "Gums lost his canteen for disobeying a screw, so he didn't have the burn. I'm sure he would have paid if he'd had the chance."

"Fucking hell," said Charlie, "how unlucky can you get?"

"Yeah," replied Owen, "Tank's not a bloke to fuck with."

"What's he done?"

"Shot a bloke in the head cause he looked at his missus," said Owen.

"Oh," replied Charlie.

"Letter. Parker," shouted the officer, sliding an envelope under the door.

Owen grabbed his letter and ripped it open.

"It's from my girlfriend," he said, staring at the script.

"How long you been with her?"

"A couple of years," answered Owen, "we've got a son. Eleven months."

Charlie read his book. Owen studied his letter. Bang-up - never gets any easier.

"Tea, lads," said Lips, opening the cell, "in about twenty minutes."

Charlie stood on the landing and studied his fellow prisoners. A bald bloke, about twenty-five, lashed with his walking stick at a black inmate. The black man swotted the stick and kept coming. Two officers guided the prisoner back to his cell. A third warden dealt with the bald inmate.

"Smith," he snapped, "fuck off. Back to your cell or you're nicked."

The bald inmate hobbled along the landing. Without the use of his stick, walking would have been a challenge too far.

Owen appeared from the cell holding his plastics.

"Fucking starving," he said.

"That bloke," said Charlie, "dodgy leg. Uses a stick. What happened to him?"

"He says he was blasted by armed police," replied Owen, "but he's known to be a liar."

"Oh."

"Just going to talk to Leo," said Owen, walking away.

Charlie wandered along the landing. He peered into each cell. Clusters of inmates smoked, laughed and chatted. Surrounded by people but very alone.

"Wish they'd hurry up and serve tea," pondered Charlie, mind wandering.

He bumped into the prisoner before he even realised someone was there.

"Sorry, mate," said Charlie, steadying the convict, "miles away."

"No problem, don't worry," replied the man, well dressed, well groomed and well spoken.

"He's not your average prisoner," thought Charlie, looking at him.

A CRY FOR EVER

"I'm Jamie," he said.

"I'm Charlie."

"Have you got long?"

"Only a month," replied Charlie, "what about you?"

"Eighteen months for fraud," answered Jamie, "helped myself to company funds."

"Oh," said Charlie.

"Been here for three weeks," said Jamie, "but I should be transferred to Ford open prison very soon."

"That'll be okay," said Charlie, "no fences, out to work, time will soon pass."

"I really hope so," replied Jamie.

"Are you banged up in cell seventeen?"

"Yes," answered Jamie, "why?"

"Do you share with a big bloke, bit tubby, long hair?"

"Tugsy," said Jamie.

"Tugsy?"

"That's what I call him," answered Jamie, "spends all night….. um…… satisfying himself."

"Oh, charming," said Charlie, "he looks familiar."

"He's been to prison loads of times," said Jamie.

"Do you know where?"

"Lewes, mostly," answered Jamie.

"That must be where I've seen him."

"Haven't had much luck with cell-mates," said Jamie.

"Why?"

"Before Tugsy," answered Jamie, "I was banged up with a bloke who kept self-harming. Lost count of the number of times he slashed his arms."

"What happened to him?"

"I think they took him to the hospital wing," answered Jamie.

"Oh," said Charlie.

"What about your cell-mate?"

"He's okay," answered Charlie, "I'm quite lucky."

Charlie and Jamie headed down the stairs and joined the queue for tea.

After tea, bang-up. Owen was writing a letter to his girlfriend, so Charlie followed his example.

"Dear Cath," he wrote, "life much as I remember……….. looking forward to getting out but time drags by……………. hope you are well……………."

He chewed his pen, trying to be witty and funny.

"Please write back," he concluded, failing miserably.

It was a long night. Past midnight, wide awake with little hope of sleep. Charlie lay on his bed, staring into the darkness. Not even a yawn. Owen snored softly. He'd been asleep since ten o'clock.

"Lucky fucker," thought Charlie, listening to the soft, regular breathing, "wish I could get to sleep so quickly."

"Woof, woof, woof, woof."

"Oh, fuck," muttered Charlie, "here we go again. Wonder how long it'll last tonight?"

The barking stopped long before Charlie fell asleep.

Morning dawned. Breakfast, bang-up. Lunch, bang-up. Canteen, two ounces of Dark Brown, two packets of Rizlas and a box of matches. Bang-up. Exercise, bang-up. Tea, bang-up. Association, final bang-up.

Charlie and Owen sat in their cell, another day closer to freedom, reading and chatting.

"What a day," said Owen, "going to get my head down."

"Okay," replied Charlie, "I'll just finish this chapter."

He lay on his bed and tried to concentrate on his book. Voices from other cells were ever present but, after a while, little more than a background noise.

"Blimey," he pondered, straining to see Owen's watch, "been reading for almost two hours. It's nearly one o'clock in the morning."

He put the book on the table, had a last roll-up, then climbed under the covers. Surprisingly, he fell asleep within minutes. Arguments raged outside the cell window long after.

Charlie stirred in his sleep. Something wasn't right. A warm, sticky sensation on his face. By the landing light, blood was visible on his arms and shirt. Adrenalin dispelled any drowsiness. He touched his face with his hand. His nose was dripping.

"It's only a fucking nose bleed," he muttered, struggling out of bed, "nothing to worry about."

He turned on the cell light. Owen slept soundly, unaware of the commotion.

"Take a nuclear bomb to wake him," pondered Charlie, squeezing the bridge of his nose and tilting back his head.

The blood kept coming. He took some toilet tissue and

covered his nose. Head back, he pressed firmly. Minutes ticked by.

"Got to stop soon," he muttered.

He looked at the watch on the table.

"Nearly four o'clock," he sighed, "only been asleep for a few hours."

Ten minutes and his neck had started to ache. He carefully removed the tissue.

"Think it's stopped," he decided, touching his face.

The white toilet tissue had been dyed a bright red. He flushed it away. Even the chain flushing failed to wake Owen. Charlie cleaned all patches of blood using a dampened tissue.

"Leukaemia! Spontaneous bleeding is a symptom of leukaemia. Remember reading the medical book."

Charlie sat on his bed and rolled a cigarette.

"Don't be stupid," he muttered, "it's only a fucking nose bleed."

He puffed his roll-up.

"If you've got leukaemia you're in trouble. You could die. What will happen to Charlotte? Or you could spend so much time having treatment you won't be able to look after her."

He puffed furiously. Smoke filled the cell. Owen slept, blissfully unaware.

"Look," he reasoned, heart thudding, breathing fast and shallow, "there are many symptoms of leukaemia. A nose bleed, without anything else, means fuck all. Probably stress."

He lay on the bed, fighting to keep control. Deep breathing and four roll-ups gave him the upper hand. It was long after five o'clock before he was convinced. A nose bleed isn't a death sentence. Charlie flicked the light and lay in the dark. It wouldn't be long before unlock and another distressing day.

"Breakfast," said Lips, "twenty minutes."

Usual routine. After a while, individual days blended into one continuous sentence.

Charlie and Jamie walked around the exercise yard.

"Any news about your transfer to Ford?"

"Haven't heard," replied Jamie, "shouldn't be much longer."

They were joined by Gary, a burglar banged up next to Jamie. Gary had been brought up in care. Next came secure units. Then young offenders' institutions. He had finally graduated to prison. Gary and Jamie were a strange pairing. Jamie, smart appearance, good education, luxury accommodation, and Gary, few chances, homemade tattoos, available squats.

"Alright, Jamie?" said Gary.

"Yes," replied Jamie, "have you met Charlie?"

"Hello, mate," said Gary, "what you in for?"

"Fight with a bloke down an alley," answered Charlie, "only got a month."

"No problem," said Gary.

"What about you?"

"Thirty months for dwellings," answered Gary, "had only been out for six weeks when I got nicked."

"Will you serve it here?"

"Not sure," replied Gary, "have to wait and see."

"Looking forward to getting out?"

"I guess," answered Gary, "but I keep getting extra days."

"Oh," said Charlie.

"Down the block, today, on governor's report," said Gary, "and the bastards gave me two weeks loss of remission."

"What for?"

"Called a woman screw a dirty whore," answered Gary.

They must have completed thirty laps of the yard.

"That's it, lads," yelled the officer on exercise duty, "inside. Wait at the gate."

Association was an expensive affair. Charlie bet four roll-ups on a game of pool. Gary proved to be an exceptional player, and retired to his cell with a healthy dose of nicotine.

Charlie and Owen sat in their cell, never struggling for conversation.

"Talking to Leo during association," said Owen.

"Oh," said Charlie.

"He was in the chapel and they were praying for some bloke who'd had a heart attack," said Owen.

"Who?"

"Not sure," replied Owen, "but I know he was on this unit."

"Bloody hell," muttered Charlie.

"Apparently," continued Owen, "the attack happened when the night screws were on duty."

"And?"

"Well," said Owen, "at first they thought he was faking."

"Blimey," whispered Charlie.

"When they realised he was genuine, they had to get the keys," said Owen.

"What do you mean?"

"Night screws don't carry keys," said Owen, "security reasons."

"Oh."

"Screw got the keys from the office and opened the cell," answered Owen.

"Is the bloke okay?"

"I heard," said Owen, "that he's critical in an outside hospital."

"Fucking hell," muttered Charlie.

Owen started writing another letter to his beloved, so Charlie picked up his book.

"If you had a heart attack you'd be dead before you got out the cell," he thought.

Charlie could feel his heart thumping against his chest.

"Look," he reasoned, breathing deeply, "it's unlikely you'll have a heart attack. You're not very old. Heart's only beating like fuck cause you're panicking. Get a grip and you'll be fine."

He sat on his bed for twenty minutes trying to control his fluctuating anxiety. He'd yet to read a full sentence.

"How old was the bloke who had the heart attack?"

"I heard," answered Owen, looking up from his letter, "he was in his fifties."

"Oh," replied Charlie, "just wondered."

He tossed his book onto the table and stretched out on his bed. His breathing and heart rate were almost normal. Anxiety was controlled……. for now!

Owen threw his pen onto the table.

"Finished," he announced.

"Good letter?"

"It'll keep her happy," replied Owen.

Charlie rolled a cigarette and offered one to Owen. They sat in the cell, smoking and chatting. Voices, outside the window, blended into the background. Crimes, women…… many topics were discussed.

"Bloody hell," said Owen, glancing at his watch, "it's past

two-thirty."

"Blimey," said Charlie.

"Better get some kip," said Owen.

"Yeah," replied Charlie.

"I'll have one more burn."

"There's something missing," said Charlie.

"Sorry?"

"I haven't heard any barking noises for the last couple of nights," said Charlie.

"Didn't I tell you?"

"Tell me what?"

"I was gabbing to Leo," answered Owen, "and he was telling me about that geezer."

"What's he say?"

"Well," replied Owen, dragging his fag, "the bloke attacked a screw. Took a chunk out his ear."

"Fucking hell," muttered Charlie.

"Anyway," continued Owen, "screws came and took him down the block."

"So, he's down the block?"

"According to Leo," said Owen, "on the way down the block, there was a struggle and geezer fell down the stairs."

"Blimey," said Charlie, "and what happened to him?"

"Well," answered Owen, "Leo reckons he's dead."

"Dead?"

"Yeah," answered Owen, "Leo heard he'd died."

"Bloody hell," muttered Charlie.

"Can't be sure he's got it right," said Owen," but geezer ain't on the unit."

"Blimey."

Owen crushed his roll-up in the ashtray and climbed into bed. Charlie turned off the light, then lay down. Within minutes, soft, regular breathing indicated Owen had dropped off.

"Lucky bugger," pondered Charlie, staring into the dark, "must have a clear conscience; nothing keeps him awake."

Charlie flipped over his pillow and tried to sleep. Body tired but mind alert.

"That poor fucker who kept barking," he pondered, "what an end. Being dragged down the block and............. nothing else."

He pulled his blanket over his face. Nothing seemed to work.

A CRY FOR EVER

"Got a bit of a headache," he thought, rubbing his forehead.

"Headache. Sure that can be a symptom of leukaemia. So, nosebleed and headache......... leukaemia."

Charlie lay in the dark, heart racing and gasping for oxygen. Agitated, restless and anxious.

"Okay," he thought, "get a grip and your heartbeat will return to normal. Then you'll be able to breathe properly."

He lay on his back, breathing deeply. It must have taken at least thirty minutes before normal service was resumed. Heartbeat and breathing felt normal. A slight tingling sensation lingered in his fingers and toes.

"Sure that's okay," he decided, shaking his hands, "just hyperventilation. Quite normal after a panic attack."

He rolled onto his front.

"Head feels like there's a little man in there with a hammer," he thought.

He buried his face in the pillow. Fighting to control further attacks of anxiety.

"Look," he pondered, "people get headaches all the time. One of the most common complaints. Definitely doesn't mean you've got leukaemia. As for the nosebleed......... stress. Bloody unlucky to get both in the same week but just a coincidence."

Charlie took the upper hand in the battle of anxiety. One battle didn't mean he'd won the war.

Another hour passed before he slipped into a restless sleep.

"He was lying in hospital....... Catherine and Charlotte........ at his bedside........ doctor................. bad news........"

He couldn't rest, even when asleep!

Following morning, business as usual. Medication. Porridge for breakfast. Bang-up. Mashed potato and liver for lunch. Bang-up. Exercise. Bang-up. Charlie sat on his bed and smoked a roll-up. Owen struggled to explain his feelings to his girlfriend in a four-page letter. Footsteps could be heard along the landing.

"Must be delivering the post," said Owen.

"Probably," replied Charlie, "it'd be nice to get a letter."

"Parker, letter. Lloyd, letter."

Charlie grabbed the two envelopes and handed Owen his letter.

"It's from my mate, Dave," said Owen, scanning the letter.

Charlie pulled out the folded piece of paper and started to read.

"It's from Catherine," he said, "the girl I've been seeing."

"Oh," said Owen, "good news?"

"Not sure yet," replied Charlie, studying the scrawl.

He started the second page.

"Bloody hell," he muttered, eyes fixed on the letter.

"Problems?"

"No," replied Charlie, "not exactly."

"What then?"

"Catherine's pregnant," answered Charlie.

"Were you trying for a baby?"

"Not exactly," replied Charlie.

"Are you pleased?"

"Yeah," replied Charlie, "reckon I am."

"Does she say anything else in the letter?"

"Says she's really pleased about it," answered Charlie.

"Well," said Owen, "that's fucking brilliant."

"Guess so," answered Charlie.

"Better celebrate with a roll-up," suggested Owen, opening his tobacco.

Charlie and Owen sat in the cell, chatting and smoking. Names were considered...... then rejected. Marriage was considered ...... then rejected. Career prospects were considered....... then rejected. Before long, a female officer unlocked the cell.

"Tea, lads," she said.

Charlie and Owen stood on the landing watching the warden unlock door after door. Other landings were manned by other officers.

"Haven't seen her before," said Charlie.

"She's been on the unit a few times," replied Owen.

"Would you?"

"Got to be joking," answered Owen, "short, fat, bigger biceps than me, cropped hair......... no fucking way."

"She is a bit dumpy," said Charlie.

"Saying that," continued Owen, "after five years....... maybe. After five years and five pints....... probably."

Tea was served and consumed in the cell.

"Disgusting," said Owen, clearing his plate, "what the fuck do they put in the pie?"

164

Association, three games of pool, six roll-ups lost on wager with Gary. Bang-up.

"Better reply to Dave," said Owen, picking up a pen and paper.

"Okay," replied Charlie, "think I'll write to Catherine and let her know how pleased I am."

Owen completed three pages, chucked his pen onto the table and rolled a cigarette. A couple of minutes, a couple of sentences and Charlie signed his name.

"Hopes she appreciates this letter," he said, opening his tobacco.

They talked for nearly an hour. A good conversationalist made bang-up so much more bearable.

"I'm shagged," said Owen, yawning, "think I'll call it a night."

Owen used the toilet, brushed his teeth and lay under the covers. Charlie finished his roll-up, got ready and curled up in his blanket. It was a matter of minutes before gentle snoring filled the cell.

"Lucky sod," thought Charlie, trying to get comfortable.

He rolled onto his front and buried his face in the pillow.

"Still life ain't all shit," he pondered, "already got one child. Now, another is on the way. Maybe, I'll stay with the mother. When I go home..... got a real chance."

He turned on his side.

"Ain't going to let OCD force me back to prison," he determined.

He rolled onto his back.

"So many reasons to stay away from trouble," he thought, "with help, reckon I'll be okay."

He lay on his back, staring at the ceiling. He rubbed his forehead. A little uncomfortable, a slight ache, minor pain.

"It's nothing," he muttered, "ignore it."

The more he worried, the worse the pain became.

"Another headache. This could be serious. Brain tumour! Leukaemia! What bastard luck....... just when the future looked so bright."

He closed his eyes, breathing deeply to control his anger and anxiety.

"Think about it," he urged, "if you worry about something, it's likely to happen. Since you've been shitting yourself about headaches....... what's happened? Every fucking night, you've got a headache. Still don't mean a brain tumour or leukaemia. It's probably nothing serious. You're going to spend your whole life worrying about something that may never happen. You've a bright future…….. for fuck's sake…… live it."

He lay still, breathing deeply, focusing on the positives. Owen snored gently……… peaceful with his predicament.

"Suppose if you ain't worried," pondered Charlie, listening to his cell-mate, "there ain't a problem. Wish I could be like that."

He pulled his blanket over his face.

"I've just got to stop these fucking ideas ruining my life," he pondered, "only going to worry about something if it actually happens."

It was almost two thirty before Charlie, excited by positive determination, dozed under his tatty blanket.

Chapter 12

The following day, Charlie and Owen started a fitness routine during afternoon bang-up. Press-ups, sit-ups and jogging on the spot passed the time. Charlie sat on his chair puffing and panting.

"You going out for exercise?"

"Yeah," replied Owen, "need some fresh air."

Charlie rolled a cigarette and handed the tobacco to Owen.

"Ta," said Owen.

The cell opened. Dumper Truck stood at the door.

"Going out for exercise, lads?"

"Yeah," said Charlie, standing up.

Owen grabbed his coat and squeezed past Dumper Truck onto the landing.

Charlie walked around the yard chatting to Jamie.

"Any news on your transfer?"

"Haven't heard anything," replied Jamie, "but it can't be much longer."

"Where's Gary today?"

"Stayed in his cell," answered Jamie, "got a bit of a headache."

They'd done at least thirty laps. Every prisoner walking in the same direction. One inmate, dressed in a long coat, decided to be different. Charlie noticed him as he strolled purposefully across the yard. Charlie nudged Jamie.

"What's he doing?"

"Not sure," replied Jamie, "but looks like he's on a mission."

"He does," agreed Charlie, watching intently.

The prisoner, a tall, bulky man, tattooed hands and cropped hair, lessened his stride. He stopped in front of another inmate. A short man, slightly built, curly hair and glasses.

"Looks like he's reached his target," muttered Charlie.

"Yeah," agreed Jamie.

"Who's the other bloke? He looks a bit weird."

"His name's Derek," answered Jamie, "think he grassed on the other prisoner."

"What for?"

"Think the big bloke was taxing him," replied Jamie, "and he went to the screws."

"Oh," said Charlie.

"Even the screws think he's a crackpot," added Jamie.

The prisoner, quick as lightening, pulled a lump of wood from inside his coat.

"Fucking hell," muttered Charlie, "where the hell did he get that from?"

"Looks like a table leg," answered Jamie.

Derek didn't move. He looked towards the wardens........ his only chance. Lips and Dumper Truck seemed oblivious to the situation. They laughed and joked, blissfully unaware. Derek covered his head with trembling hands waiting for the inevitable onslaught. He didn't wait long. The wood, swung for his head, smashed both his hands. He shrieked and tumbled to the floor. Other prisoners backed away. Two more hammer blows across the back.

"Bloody hell," murmured Charlie, "a direct hit to the head would kill him."

"This is horrible," whispered Jamie.

Derek yelped as the wood shattered a kneecap. Lips looked towards the melee, nudged Dumper Truck and walked across the yard.

"Screws have realised," said Jamie, "about time."

"Not exactly hurrying," said Charlie, "it'll be a murder if they're not careful."

"I know," answered Jamie.

"Last time I was here," muttered Charlie to Jamie, "another weird geezer got a hiding. Screws didn't seem to care."

Lips and Dumper Truck ambled casually; could have been enjoying a moonlight stroll along the beach.

The prisoner wielded the wood. It was a frenzied attack with no thought of the consequences. Two more lashes across Derek's back. His head jerked, his face cracking against the concrete. His glasses shattered, his nose broke, his teeth cracked.

Lips and Dumper Truck stepped up the pace, finally aware of the serious nature of the incident.

"Oi," shouted Lips, "what the fuck's going on?"

The prisoner, happy with his work, handed the table leg to Lips.

Everything happened quickly. Two medics tended to Derek. They quickly realised the severity of his injuries and he was carried from the yard on a stretcher.

His assailant was led to the gate, back on the unit, then straight down the block. A warden, white suit, mask and gloves, cleaned the blood. The other prisoners, queued at the gate, filed onto the unit, then bang-up until tea.

Charlie sat on his bed, puffed a cigarette, chatting to Owen.
"Exercise was fucking crazy," said Charlie.
"You know it," replied Owen.
"Do you know the geezer with the wood?"
"I've heard about him," answered Owen, "bit of a psycho. He's been taking Derek's canteen every week."
"Oh," said Charlie.
"Anyway," continued Owen, "Derek broke a major rule....... he grassed him."
"What happened?"
"Geezer got seven days down the block and lost a month," replied Owen.
"Oh," said Charlie, "that explains it."
"Grassing someone like that is serious," said Owen, "he's going to be inside for years so he ain't got nothing to lose."
"What's he in for?"
"Security van, firing at police to resist arrest, supplying drugs."
"Blimey," murmured Charlie.

Tea time. Cell opened. Queued at the gate. Collected meal. Stomached lean cuisine. Banged up until association. Two roll-ups earned during association. Banged up for the night. Charlie chatted to Owen for a couple of hours until his cellmate fell asleep. It was the early hours of the morning before Charlie dropped off.

"Breakfast, lads," said Dumper Truck, opening the door, "served in about ten minutes."
Charlie fell out his pit, collected his medication and waited at the gate. First in the queue for breakfast, might not be cold. A bowl of porridge, then bang-up. A letter to Catherine passed an hour. Unlock.
"Going to have a shower," said Charlie, grabbing his towel.
"Okay," replied Owen, "see you later."
Charlie wandered along the landing and peered into the shower block.
"Good," he thought, "it's empty. Bit of peace."
He chose a shower and checked the temperature.
"Perfect," he muttered, as the water touched his hand.

He unclipped his dungaree strap. The door opened - Tugsy.

"Oh, fuck it," thought Charlie, "what a wank."

Tugsy walked into the block. No towel, just a big grin.

"Hello," leered Tugsy, "trying to wash away the smell of piss?"

"Sorry?"

"Has any piss been tipped over you?"

"Not today," replied Charlie, "lucky me."

Charlie stopped undressing and stared at the ground. Trouble was always best avoided, especially with only a few days until release. Tugsy had other ideas. He wanted a reaction.

"Do you drink piss as well as wash in it?"

"I'm going," said Charlie, fastening his strap.

"You're full of shit, you fucking prick," sneered Tugsy.

Charlie hesitated.

"I can't ignore this," he thought, "I won't survive another day."

"Arsehole," mocked Tugsy.

Reluctantly, Charlie walked towards Tugsy.

"Leave it out or I'll do ya," he mumbled.

"Suck my dick," replied Tugsy, mockingly.

Charlie, two-handed, pushed against Tugsy's chest. The prisoner stepped backwards to maintain balance. Tugsy whipped a right hook. Sharp, powerful and accurate. Charlie's mouth bled. He felt dizzy but didn't go down. Head bowed, he lashed with his left. A jab, very weak and little precision, brushed Tugsy's cheek.

"He's going to fucking kill me," panicked Charlie, stumbling forward.

He grabbed Tugsy and, head pressed into his chest, clung on. Tugsy struggled violently. If he freed his arms, he'd be able to do so much damage.

"Fucking hang on," urged Charlie, praying for a miracle.

He was aware of movement. The door of the shower block had opened. Maybe, just maybe, miracles do happen. Even in prison.

"What the fuck's going on?"

"Gary," thought Charlie, recognising the voice, "an angel in disguise."

"You okay, Charlie?"

Tugsy stopped struggling. Not impressed with the odds, retreat with dignity was the best option. Charlie released his grip, stepped backwards and stood watching Tugsy.

"Don't want to give him an opening," thought Charlie, "a second….. that's all it takes."

Tugsy stared at Charlie, then at Gary.

"Get fucked," he snarled, "nothing for me in here."

"That's right," said Gary, "now fuck off."

Tugsy barged past Charlie and stomped out of the showers.

"What a cock," said Gary, "you okay?"

"Good," answered Charlie, "glad to see you."

"No problem," said Gary.

"Anyway, thanks," said Charlie, "could have got a bit of a hiding."

"Lip looks sore," said Gary.

"It's okay," replied Charlie, "I'll clean it and it'll hardly show."

They left the showers. Charlie went to his cell, cleaned his face, then joined the queue for lunch. Liver, bacon, potatoes and peas, then bang-up.

"Your mouth looks a bit swollen," said Owen.

"It's not too bad," replied Charlie, "bit of a tussle with geezer banged up along the landing."

"Oh," said Owen, "anyone I know?"

"Doubt it," answered Charlie.

"Need any back-up?"

"No," replied Charlie, "it's sorted."

"Okay, then," said Owen.

Owen wrote a letter and Charlie lay on his bed listening to the radio.

"Exercise," said Dumper Truck, opening the cell, "are you going out?"

Charlie and Owen stood up. Actions speak louder than words.

Charlie circled the yard with Jamie and Gary.

"I hate this place," said Jamie, "can't wait to go."

"Know what you mean," replied Charlie, "any date for transfer?"

"As far as I know it'll be next Wednesday," answered Jamie.

"That's good," said Charlie.

"Yeah," said Jamie, "apparently they give you a train ticket and you go there on trust."

"Do a runner," suggested Gary, "I would."

"No chance," replied Jamie, "I'm going to behave myself, do my time and never come back."

Sixty-two laps in one hour.

"Wait at the gate," yelled Dumper Truck, "time for bang-up."

Charlie walked along the landing and stood outside the cell. A couple of minutes later, he was joined by Owen.

"Screw not opened the door?"

"Not yet," answered Charlie, "think it takes her a long time to climb the stairs."

"Not surprised," said Owen, "bit chubby."

Dumper Truck wheezed along the landing. Lips was busy at the other end. She unlocked the door.

"There you are, lads," she said.

"You dirty whore!"

Charlie, anxiety rising, clenched his teeth and covered his mouth. With heart racing and breathing shallow and rapid, he leaned against the wall. Talking wasn't on the agenda, standing being an almighty challenge.

"Thanks," said Owen, walking into the cell.

Charlie followed his cell-mate and flopped onto the bed. A sickly feeling of hopelessness. He struggled to regulate his breathing. Beads of perspiration prickled on his forehead. He replayed the incident inside his mind, again and again. He failed to notice Owen's puzzled expression.

"You okay, Charlie?"

"Fine," replied Charlie, "just feel a bit sick and bit of a headache."

"Have a sleep, mate," said Owen.

"I'll just lie on my bed," replied Charlie.

Owen picked up his book and started to read. Charlie lay on the bed, eyes fixed on the ceiling, trying to make sense of the situation.

"You didn't say a word," he pondered, "if you had called her a dirty whore then she'd have nicked you."

He rolled onto his front.

"What if she comes back and nicks you? You'll be on governor's report. You'll lose a couple of weeks so you'll serve the full month. Not much use to Charlotte."

Charlie sat up, rolled a cigarette and puffed furiously.

"Get control," he urged, "you didn't say anything. It's just a bloody worry. Anyway, who gives a fuck about two extra weeks?"

Smoke filled the cell.

"If you did say something, then you could have acted on other intrusions."

He crushed his roll-up in the ashtray, then rolled another.

"Look," he thought, "I didn't say anything. It was just an intrusion, a worry. I didn't act upon it........ never have and never would!"

Twenty minutes passed, breathing and heart rate were almost normal. Charlie kept replaying the situation in his mind. Owen studied the text in his paperback. Charlie glanced at Owen, desperate to check the worry.

"When the fat screw opened the door," said Charlie, "did I say anything?"

"Like what?"

"Anything you'd consider strange," said Charlie.

"Not that I remember," answered Owen, "why do you ask?"

"No reason," answered Charlie.

Owen turned the page and kept reading. Charlie lay on his bed and kept thinking.

"Still worrying," pondered Charlie, struggling with anger and anxiety.

Charlie rolled onto his front.

"What the fuck have I done to deserve this shit?"

He buried his head in his pillow.

"When she opens for tea," he decided, "I'll try and talk to her."

Thirty minutes passed.

"Tea, lads," said Lips, opening the door.

"Fuck," thought Charlie, "where's Dumper Truck?"

He marched along the landing, head bowed, miles away. He didn't notice Tugsy until he walked into him.

"Just fuck yourself, cock sucker," spat Charlie, "or I swear, I'll kill you."

Tugsy looked shocked, almost dumbfounded. He glared at Charlie, muttered under his breath, and kept walking.

Charlie paced along the landing, down the stairs and......... bingo. Dumper Truck was chatting to a black inmate on the ground floor.

Charlie paced across the floor and hovered by Dumper Truck. She seemed engrossed in her discussion with the tall, black prisoner. It sounded like they were debating the effect of a good prison report on a Crown Court judge.

"It's now or never," pondered Charlie, "a chance to stop

worrying."

He stood close, hands in pockets, desperate for his opportunity.

"A good report from a prison officer can reduce your sentence by a third," said Dumper Truck.

"Hope so," said the prisoner.

"Hurry up, for fuck's sake," pondered Charlie, "I look such a prick, standing here."

Charlie took his tobacco from his pocket and rolled a cigarette.

"Better go and get my plastics," said the prisoner, "it won't be long 'til tea."

"Okay," replied Dumper Truck, "and, remember, behave yourself."

The prisoner turned and walked away.

"Miss," said Charlie, stepping forward.

"Yes," she answered.

"Have you got a light?"

"Of course," she replied, handing Charlie a lighter, "here you are."

"Brilliant," thought Charlie, taking the lighter, "she's fine. You don't behave like that if someone's called you a dirty whore."

He lit his roll-up and returned the lighter.

"Thanks, Miss," he said.

"No problem," she answered, flashing a lovely smile.

He turned and walked towards the stairs.

"Pucker," he thought, deliriously happy, "worry over."

He climbed the stairs.

"She ain't much to look at," he pondered, "but full marks for personality. And……. what a smile."

He grabbed his plastics from the cell and waited at the gate.

The last few days passed quickly without much incident. A couple of headaches caused minor concerns. Normal anxiety levels were quickly resumed. The last night, banged up after association, Charlie lay on his bed chatting to Owen.

"Looking forward to going home?"

"Yeah," replied Charlie, "can't wait to see Charlotte. And it'll be good to see Catherine. Hope things are okay with the pregnancy."

"Sure they are," said Owen, "they'd have got a message to you if there'd been any problems."

"I suppose," answered Charlie.

"So," asked Owen, "will you get wrecked tomorrow night?"

"Doubt it," answered Charlie, "probably get Catherine to come round and we'll look after Charlotte."

"Fucking hell," said Owen, "when I get out....... booze.......all night...... see my woman...... it's going to be the best."

Charlie rolled a cigarette and dragged slowly.

"It's my son's birthday in a few weeks," said Owen.

"Oh," replied Charlie, "he'll be one, won't he?"

"Yeah," answered Owen, "just hope I'm out of here by the time he's five."

"You should be," said Charlie.

"Possible," answered Owen, "but if I'm found guilty could get ten."

"Any chance of not guilty?"

"Solicitor doesn't reckon I've a hope in hell," replied Owen.

"Oh," said Charlie, "best to plead guilty and have good mitigation."

"That's what I'll do."

Two hours passed. Bang-up was much easier with an end in sight.

"Better get some sleep," said Owen, snuggling under his blanket, "wake me in the morning before you go."

"Will do," replied Charlie, "sleep well."

Charlie lay on his bed, staring at the ceiling. It was only a matter of minutes before soft snores filled the cell.

"I wish I could sleep so quickly," pondered Charlie, glancing across the pad, "it'd make bang-up so fucking easy."

Charlie rolled onto his front.

"A new start tomorrow," he mused, "back with Tiger. Catherine's pregnant. No criminal charges. Intrusions are bad but I've so many reasons to beat them."

He tossed and turned, nervously excited at the prospect of freedom. Owen slept, like a baby, unfazed by his future. Long after three o'clock, long after voices outside fell silent, Charlie finally dozed.

"Lloyd, get your stuff ready," said the officer outside the cell, "you'll be opened up in about ten minutes."

"Okay," replied Charlie, leaping out of bed, "won't be long."

Charlie pulled on his dungarees and fastened the straps. Then he folded his bedclothes and packed a few belongings.

"Owen," he hissed, "'I'm going in a minute."

"Okay, mate," murmured Owen, rolling over, "be lucky."

"I'll write to you in a few days," said Charlie.

"Yeah," muttered Owen, "don't forget."

"I don't need my tobacco," said Charlie, "so I'll leave an ounce."

Charlie tossed the tobacco onto Owen's bed.

"Thanks, mate," said Owen.

Charlie stood at the door. He could hear the warden walking along the landing, stopping, occasionally, to unlock a cell.

"People in court, people getting out," pondered Charlie, listening to the approaching footsteps, "and people being transferred."

"Go and wait at the gate," said the officer, unlocking the door, "and you'll be taken to reception."

Charlie left his cell and hurried along the landing. He knocked on a cell door.

"Jamie," he hissed, "wake up."

No response.

"Jamie, come on," he repeated, "I ain't got long."

"What?"

"I'm going now," said Charlie, "just come to say goodbye."

"Good luck, mate," muttered Jamie, "hope everything works out."

"Sure it will," replied Charlie, "good luck at Ford."

"Thanks," said Jamie, "at least I won't be here much longer."

"See ya," said Charlie, "keep out of trouble."

Charlie left Jamie and hurried along the landing. He banged on another cell.

"Gary," he hissed, "just come to wish you well. I'm going."

"You know the score," mumbled Gary, "you've been here before. You know the crack, you're coming back."

"Hope not," said Charlie.

"Just don't get caught," answered Gary.

"Do my best," said Charlie.

"Good luck, mate," said Gary, "have a pint for me."

"See you," said Charlie.

He walked to the gate and stood with all the other prisoners leaving that morning. Some were off to court. The vast majority would be back that evening. Some were being transferred to other prisons. Open prisons for non-violent offenders, with a relaxed regime. Bang-up for violent inmates doing a long stretch. A minority were being released. How long would it be before a return to custody? Statistically, unfavourable odds.

Charlie, breakfast wasted and formalities completed, sat in the cage waiting for release. Another inmate, Alan, had also paid his debt to society.

"How long you done?"

"Only a couple of weeks," replied Charlie, "what about you?"

"Nine months," answered Alan.

"What for?"

"Attacked my neighbour with a baseball bat," replied Alan.

"Oh," said Charlie.

"We'd been feuding for years," said Alan, "and I just snapped."

Two inmates were taken from another cage, handcuffed together, and led to a van. There were already four pairs of prisoners squashed in the vehicle. A day in court...... hardly a picnic at the seaside.

The warden unlocked the cage.

"Come on, lads," he said, "let's get rid of you."

Alan and Charlie followed the warden out of reception. A hundred yards from the building to the gates. They walked through the prison grounds, with the officer in attendance. A van drove past. Eight inmates, fate in the balance, and two wardens, all peered through the barred windows. The gates slowly opened...... the grinding sound determining someone's liberty. Ten yards from the open gates. The warden stopped walking. Ex-convicts could be trusted now.

"Good luck, lads," said the warden.

Alan and Charlie walked through the gates. Sweet freedom.

"There's my wife," said Alan, pointing at a car parked on the road, "can't wait to get home."

"All the best," said Charlie.

Alan rushed to the car, opened the door and climbed inside.

"Steady bird," thought Charlie, "nice bloke. Never know, might be his last visit."

He gazed across the fields. Grass, trees and bushes, as far as the eye could see. One road led to the prison, crossing the countryside. The huge car park and secure buildings were a separate world. A world to be left behind, gone but never forgotten.

Charlie stood at the side of the road, enjoying the breeze on his face.

"Hope Lucy gets here soon," he pondered, "she definitely said, in her letter, she wouldn't be late."

He paced along the road, turned, and paced back.

"I'm free," he thought, "first day of the rest of my life. Tiger, Catherine, new baby...... it's going to be pucker."

He looked into the distance. A lady, Yorkshire Terrier on a lead, shuffled across the field. Every five or six yards, she stumbled on the uneven ground.

"Poor old thing," thought Charlie, "she must have walked miles. There's no houses nearby."

"You haven't hurt her, have you?"

Charlie felt a little uneasy. Heart rate increased and breathing became shallow.

"Don't be so bloody stupid," he cursed, "she's about fifty yards away and hasn't walked anywhere near."

Controlling his anxiety was quick and efficient. The idea stimulated by the intrusion hadn't been severe. Anxiety levels were back to normal within minutes. A slight headache, depression and anger were lasting casualties.

"My body is free," thought Charlie, "but as far as my mind..... I'm doing a life sentence."

Lucy parked near her brother. This new beginning had turned into a haze of OCD. Charlie clambered into the car, leaving prison behind, but taking his false friend along for the ride.

Chapter 13

Days passed in a blur. Catherine moved in with Charlie as soon as she took maternity leave from work. Scans showed a healthy baby. Catherine opted to keep the baby's gender a surprise.

It was a clear, bright Tuesday. Charlie, Charlotte, Catherine and 'bump' were watching Jungle Book in the lounge.

"I'm really tired," yawned Catherine, "think I'll have a sleep."

"Okay," said Charlie, "see you when you wake up."

Catherine climbed off the sofa and trudged out the lounge.

"Do you want to go to the park, Tiger?"

"Yes," replied Charlotte.

"Okay," said Charlie, "let's get ready."

He locked the back door from the inside, leaving the key in the lock. He took his front door key from a drawer and walked into the hall.

"See you later," he called to Catherine, "we're just going to the park."

"Okay," she replied, "have a good time."

Charlotte walked into the hall, sensibly dressed for a chilly day.

"Come on, then, Tiger," said Charlie, "let's get going."

He open the door, gasping as the icy air rushed against his face.

"Glad you've worn a hat, Tiger," he said, "it's very cold for the time of year."

"Hat and gloves," answered Charlotte.

Charlie checked he had the right key, shoved it into his pocket and slammed the door. He took Charlotte's hand and walked down the drive.

"Are you sure you shut the door?"

Five or six more paces. Each step shorter than the step before.

"Course I did," he thought, "I slammed it so hard it nearly broke."

Three or four more paces. Each slightly more hesitant than the previous.

"What if you forgot? Catherine is sleeping in the house. No-one else is there. She's pregnant. What if something happened?"

Charlie stopped walking. He stood in the driveway, holding

Charlotte's hand.

"I know I shut the door," he thought, "I'd swear to it."

He stood still. A major decision had to be taken.

"Is it worth taking such a big risk?"

He turned and walked back to the house.

"Just got to check I've shut the door, Tiger," he said, "don't want someone to go in and give Catherine a nasty surprise."

He pulled against the door.

"Definitely shut," he said.

Back down the drive…….. ten paces before doubts began again.

"What if you didn't check the door properly? Are you sure you didn't open it?"

Two stuttering paces.

"Bollocks," thought Charlie, "this is bloody ridiculous. The door was definitely closed. Course I didn't open it."

He stopped, still holding Charlotte's hand.

"It'd be quicker just to check. You'll only worry, if you don't."

Charlie turned and headed back. He pulled the door.

"Shut," he said.

He pulled again.

"Definitely shut."

One step down the drive. Turned round, stepped back and tugged the door.

"The door is closed," he stated.

He put his hand in the letterbox. You couldn't get a better grip on a closed door. He tugged again.

"There is no way anyone could get through this door without a crowbar," he muttered.

Charlotte held Charlie's other hand, bemused by her father's strange behaviour.

Charlie slid his hand from the letterbox. The door slammed shut. He gripped the Yale lock. Another pull. Slight movement, confirming the door was closed and could only be opened with the key.

"Safe as houses, Tiger," he said, "we'd better get going."

"Yes," replied Charlotte.

They walked down the drive. Charlie struggled with a few lingering doubts. Anxiety levels were slightly high as he turned into the road. By the time they arrived at the swings, any doubts had been dispelled. Apart from a niggling headache, Charlie escaped relatively unscathed.

"So," he said, pushing the swing, "are you looking forward to getting a new playmate?"

"Think so, " answered Charlotte.

"That's good," said Charlie, "would you like a little brother or sister?"

"Sister," replied Charlotte.

An elderly couple passed the park enclosure. Charlie watched the lady, slightly anxious. He kept her under observation until she disappeared behind the clubhouse.

"She's fine," thought Charlie, "nothing happened. No worries."

Charlie pushed the swing a little higher. Charlotte giggled and held on a little tighter.

"Where's the baby now?"

"In Catherine's tummy," answered Charlie.

"Who put it there?"

"Look at the doggy by the tree," said Charlie, pointing at an ugly mutt with his leg cocked, "what a beautiful doggy."

"Yes," said Charlotte.

"Do you want to have a go on the slide?"

"Yes," answered Charlotte.

An hour on the slide, then a slow walk home. Charlie stood at the front door and pulled his key from his pocket.

"The door is shut," he pondered, turning the key, "didn't have anything to worry about."

Catherine's 'bump' grew day by day. Where were the weeks going? Charlie really enjoyed living with Catherine and watching a new life developing inside her. It was after nine o'clock on a Wednesday evening. The day had been spent playing in the woods. Charlotte, completely exhausted, slept soundly in her bed. Charlie and Catherine, slumped on the sofa, were watching Scum on video.

"Any ideas for names?" asked Catherine.

"Yes," replied Charlie.

"Oh?"

"If it's a boy," said Charlie, "I'd love to call him Colin."

"Oh," said Catherine, "are you sure?"

"Definite," replied Charlie, "no doubt about it."

"What about a girl?"

"Not sure," answered Charlie, "what do you think?"

"I quite like Emily or Lauren," answered Catherine.

"Oh," said Charlie, "I prefer Chloe or Chelsea."

"Don't know," said Catherine.

Charlie stood up.

"Just going outside for a fag," he said.

He walked out of the back door. This was the least he could do to help Catherine win her battle with nicotine addiction. He puffed away in the garden. It was a cold, dark night.

"They say smoking kills," pondered Charlie, "if I have to keep coming outside it'll be pneumonia that does for me."

He walked back into the lounge. Catherine was struggling to stay awake.

"Got an idea," said Charlie, sitting down, "what about Caroline?"

"Caroline?"

"Yeah," answered Charlie, "my best friend at school was called Caroline."

"Well," said Catherine, "I suppose it's a possibility."

A young inmate was bent over in the green-house.

"This is a horrible film," said Catherine, averting her gaze, "I'm going to bed."

"Okay," said Charlie, "I won't be long."

Charlie watched the same inmate slash his wrists.

A car parked outside the house.

"Must be Hazel and Lucy," decided Charlie, "back from visiting a friend in hospital.

Hazel and Lucy walked into the kitchen, quick cup of tea, brief catch-up with Charlie, then off to bed. Early start in the morning.

Charlie switched off the television and video. Then he checked the front door was closed and the back door was locked. He pressed the handle and pulled the back door... just to be sure.

He cleaned his teeth, had a wash, then crept into the bedroom. Catherine snored softly... being pregnant was very tiring. Charlie climbed on the bed, doing his best not to disturb his sleeping girlfriend. He lay on his back and stared at the ceiling.

"Are you sure the back door was locked? What if there's an intruder in the night?"

Charlie, carefully, rolled onto his stomach.

"Get a grip," he muttered, "you checked the back door. It

was locked."

"Can you be absolutely certain?"

Charlie buried his face into the pillow.

"I know I checked the door," he mumbled, "I'd stake my life on it."

"Is it worth the risk? Why don't you check?"

Charlie climbed from his pit, frustrated at his lack of self-belief. He checked the back door. Surprise, surprise..... it was locked. He returned to bed.

"You sure it was locked? You didn't open it?"

He rolled over and tried to relax. No chance. He tried to ignore the niggling doubts. No chance.

"What if you opened the door? What if something happened? Charlotte's in her room and Catherine is pregnant."

Charlie, agitated, struggled from his bed. He tugged the back door. It was locked. Turned away. Walked a few paces. Stopped and turned. Back to the door. Tugged harder. Still locked.

"Okay," he thought, "the door is definitely locked."

He pressed the handle and pulled. Still locked. He was agitated when checking, but anxious without checking. A final check. The door was locked. It couldn't be opened without the key. A quick glance confirmed the key was in the lock on the inside. An intruder would have to force the door or find another entry point. Whatever happened, Charlie wouldn't be at fault. He stepped away from the door.

"Definitely locked," he stated.

He went back to bed, anxiety levels almost normal. It was agitation and frustration keeping him awake until the early hours. Each day was a step closer to a new life. But each day was also tainted by obsessions and compulsions. Was the door locked? Have I got a brain tumour? Did I hurt the old lady by the tree? It was a Tuesday afternoon, around four o'clock, and Charlie sat in the consulting room chatting to Dr. King. Charlotte, Catherine and 'bump' sat with the other patients in the waiting area.

"How are things?"

"Okay," replied Charlie.

"Any major problems?"

"Well," answered Charlie, "I've spent ages checking doors."

"Explain," said Dr. king.

"When I leave the house or go to bed," replied Charlie, "I'm constantly worrying I've left the door unlocked. I have to go back and keep checking. If I don't, I can't stop worrying."

"I see," said Dr. King, "anything else?"

"I still worry if I walk past an old woman," replied Charlie, "and every little symptom means I'm dying."

"So," said Dr. King, "daily living is still difficult."

"Yeah," answered Charlie.

"Newest problem," said the psychiatrist, "checking doors."

"Yes," replied Charlie.

"Have you tried to resist the urge to check more than once?"

"I have," answered Charlie, "but if I don't do it, then I can't stop worrying."

"My advice," said Dr. King, "would be to resist as long as possible. Try and extend the time."

"I'll try," replied Charlie.

"You have to take chances," said Dr. King, "if you want to beat this. You'll see that once is enough. Accept the anxiety, resist checking and, eventually, anxiety levels will be lower in the same situation."

"I'll do my best," replied Charlie, doubtfully.

"If you resist the urge to check," repeated the doctor, "this'll prove there's no need to do it."

"Okay," said Charlie.

"Are you still taking the medication?"

"Yeah," answered Charlie, "dread to think how I'd manage without it."

"We won't reduce the amount," said Dr. King, "but you can't keep taking it indefinitely."

"Oh," muttered Charlie.

"Stay with it for now," said Dr. King.

"Thank-you," said Charlie.

"Anything else bothering you?"

"Getting loads of headaches," answered Charlie, "worry about a brain tumour or leukaemia."

"Highly unlikely," stated Dr. King, "the most common cause for headaches is stress. Wouldn't you agree that's the most likely explanation?"

"I suppose so," answered Charlie.

"Your young lady," said Dr. King, "outside in the waiting area. Is she pregnant?"

"She is," answered Charlie.

"Congratulations," said Dr. King, "I gather it was planned."

"Yeah," replied Charlie, "we're thrilled."

"Could you have a better incentive to conquer your obsessions?"

"No," replied Charlie, "I can't think of one."

"Work on it," concluded Dr. King, "and I'll see you next week."

""Thank-you," replied Charlie, standing up, "I will."

The pregnancy proved straightforward with no major complications. However, hot days during the summer were long and draining for Catherine . A Saturday evening, mid-September, and the expectant couple were home alone. Hazel was visiting a friend, just discharged from hospital. Lucy had a date: a new conquest, hardly ever mentioned. Charlotte, as usual, was staying with Linda. Catherine and Charlie sat at the kitchen table, drinking coffee.

"I really miss having a cigarette with a cup of coffee," said Catherine.

"I bet," replied Charlie, "are you going to start again after the birth?"

"I hope not," answered Catherine, "I mean I've lasted nearly seven months. It would be a shame to waste all that effort."

"Best of luck," said Charlie.

Catherine took a sip from her cup.

"Sorry to do this," said Charlie, "but just going to pop outside for a fag."

He stood up and walked to the door. A few minutes later, he was back inside. A cold evening lessened the enjoyment of a nicotine fix.

"Another cup of coffee?"

"Yes," answered Catherine, "better be the last one or I'll never get to sleep."

"Okay," said Charlie, pouring the drinks.

He handed a cup to Catherine and sat at the table.

"Going to see the midwife next week," said Catherine, taking a sip.

"Everything's okay?"

"Oh yes," replied Catherine, "just routine."

Twenty minutes and the two coffee cups were empty.

"I'm so tired," yawned Catherine, "think I'll turn-in."

"Okay," replied Charlie, "I'll just have a fag, tidy up and I'll join you."

A car parked in the drive. Minutes later, Hazel walked into the kitchen.

"Hi," said Charlie, "how's Ivy?"

"Much better," replied Hazel, "won't be long 'til she's up and about."

"That's good," said Charlie.

"I'm going to bed," said Hazel, "I feel exhausted. Ivy is quite demanding."

"Goodnight," said Charlie.

As soon as Hazel disappeared into her room, another car parked outside the house. Seconds later, Lucy opened the door.

"Hi," she said.

"Hello," replied Charlie," did you have a good evening?"

"Really nice," answered Lucy, "but I'm feeling the pace."

"Oh," said Charlie, "are you going to have a coffee?"

"No," replied Lucy, "going straight to bed."

"Okay," said Charlie, "see you in the morning."

Charlie had a roll-up, washed a couple of cups, locked the back door, used the bathroom and went to bed. Catherine already asleep, snored gently.

"At least the coffee didn't keep you awake," murmured Charlie.

He climbed into bed, taking great care not to disturb Catherine. Lying in the dark, he tried to empty his mind. Easier said than done.

"Did you lock the back door? What if you forgot?"

He rolled over.

"Think about it," he reasoned, "remember what Dr. King told you to do. Resist the urge to check."

He buried his head in the pillow, trying to keep a lid on rising anxiety.

"Got to take a risk," he urged, "eventually anxiety will drop."

He nearly managed five minutes.

"Bollocks," he hissed, climbing out his pit, "if I don't check the bloody door, I'll only lie here and worry about it."

He strode into the kitchen. The backdoor was locked. Back to bed.

It took almost fifty minutes and fifteen checks before he was satisfied the back door was locked. Agitated at his continued need for reassurance, he lay in the dark. It was another couple of hours before he finally fell asleep.

A CRY FOR EVER

The time before the birth got shorter, and 'bump' got bigger. Charlie and Charlotte spent a sunny Tuesday playing at the park. Catherine had an appointment with the midwife, preferring to go alone. At nine o'clock that evening, Charlotte slept soundly, dreaming of the swings and slide. Lucy had another date. Same escort, different venue. Hazel was dining with an old friend. Charlie and Catherine were slumped on the sofa in the lounge. Grease played on the video.

"Everything okay with the midwife?"

"Yes," replied Catherine, "baby's fine."

"Brilliant," said Charlie.

"But," continued Catherine, "baby's breech."

"Oh," said Charlie.

"That means," continued Catherine, "baby's upside down."

"Oh."

"And," continued Catherine, "because my pelvic girdle is small and baby is quite big there's no chance of baby turning."

"Okay," said Charlie.

"So," said Catherine, "baby is going to be delivered by Caesarean section."

"Oh," said Charlie, "when will that be?"

"Well," said Catherine, "they have to choose a date before baby's due so I don't go into labour."

"Right," said Charlie," have they made a decision?"

"Seventh of November," answered Catherine, "it's a Tuesday."

"Brilliant," said Charlie, "are you okay with it?"

"I suppose so," answered Catherine, "I'll have an epidural so I won't feel anything."

"And," said Charlie, "you won't have to push."

It was nearly midnight. Hazel and Lucy were still out.

"I'm exhausted," said Catherine, "time for bed."

"Okay," replied Charlie, "I'm tired as well. If I go to bed I'll have to leave the back door unlocked for Hazel and Lucy."

"That'll be fine," said Catherine.

They lay in bed. Within minutes, Catherine slept peacefully. Charlie lay awake, listening for a car outside the house. Minutes later, a car parked. He heard footsteps in the kitchen.

"Must be Hazel," he decided, "now let's hope Lucy's not

long."

It was over two hours before Lucy's car stopped in the driveway.

"About bloody time," thought Charlie, listening intently.

He heard his sister close the back door. Then there was the unmistakeable sound of the key turning in the lock.

"Thank fuck," thought Charlie, "no worries."

At peace with the world, Charlie quickly fell asleep.

Then there was the countdown to the seventh of November. A matter of weeks until the start of a new life. Tuesday had been spent at the park. An early tea, Jungle Book and Charlotte was showing classic signs of tiredness. Little resistance to bed by seven-thirty. Gently snoring ten minutes later. Charlie and Catherine flopped at the kitchen table. Lucy and Hazel, late-night shopping, shouldn't be long.

"I'm so tired," said Catherine, "carrying an extra person takes all my energy."

"Bet it does," replied Charlie.

Charlie made two cups of coffee.

"While it's quiet," he said, "I'll phone Anna and see if she can take us to the hospital."

"Okay," replied Catherine, "think I'll have a quick soak."

She headed in the direction of the bathroom. Charlie walked into the lounge, picked up the phone and dialed Anna's number.

"Hello," said Anna.

"Hi," said Charlie, "how are you?"

"Fine," replied Anna, "life's been fun."

"Yeah?"

"Not working at the moment," said Anna, "thinking about going back to college."

"Why not?"

"And," said Anna, "I've met someone."

"Who?"

"A chap called Sam," replied Anna.

"What's he like?"

"Well," answered Anna, "he's an artist. Very posh. You'd think he earns at least fifty grand a year."

"Does he?"

"No chance," replied Anna, "hardly ever works. Usually broke."

"Oh," said Charlie, "good looking?"

"Not really," replied Anna, "he's very skinny. Looks a bit of a wimp."

"Oh," said Charlie, "sounds good."

"He's very athletic between the sheets," said Anna, "certainly has lots of experience."

"Oh," said Charlie.

"Suppose," said Anna," that's the advantage of an older man."

"Suppose it is," replied Charlie, "how old is he?"

"Forty-eight," replied Anna.

"Forty-eight?"

"That's right," answered Anna.

"You're only twenty-three," said Charlie.

"I've always gone for the older man," replied Anna.

"Why not?"

"My brother is working at the same place, living with his girlfriend and drinking every night," said Anna.

"Oh," answered Charlie, "Lucy's working for the same company and goes out most evenings with her new bloke."

"How's Hazel?"

"She's fine," answered Charlie, "very busy."

"And Catherine….. how's the pregnancy?"

"Fine," replied Charlie, "baby is breech so we're booked for a Caesarean on the seventh of November."

"Right," said Anna," that's good."

"What I wanted to ask you," said Charlie, "any chance of a lift to the hospital?"

"November the seventh?"

"Yeah," confirmed Charlie.

"What time?"

"You'd need to be here before eight o'clock," answered Charlie.

"Yes," said Anna, "I'm sure that'll be fine."

"Great," said Charlie, "thanks."

Charlie hung up, stood quickly, causing slight dizziness, and walked into the kitchen.

"You almost fainted. MS. Brain tumour. You could be very ill."

"Don't be so bloody daft," urged Charlie, slumping at the table, heart thudding, "that's highly unlikely."

"But possible. Wouldn't be much use to Charlotte or new baby. What a waste of space. More of a burden than a father."

Charlie, head in hands, took deep breaths. Ten minutes later, and anxiety levels were practically normal. Blurred vision and pounding head would be relieved by a good night's sleep.

"Think about it," he urged, "be realistic. Most people feel dizzy when they stand up too quickly. Worse case scenario….. blood sugar level low. Most likely, nothing to worry about."

Charlie had just finished another cup of coffee. Headache and visual disturbances were accompanied by tingling sensations in fingers and toes and a feeling of utter hopelessness and annoyance. Catherine, fresh from her bath, sipped a hot chocolate. She noted the change of personality of Charlie.

"Are you okay?"

"Fine," lied Charlie, "bit of a headache."

"You seem really distant," said Catherine, "was Anna okay?"

"Yeah, she's fine," replied Charlie, "and she can take us to the hospital."

"That's good," said Catherine.

A car parked in the driveway. Minutes later, Hazel and Lucy struggled into the kitchen laden with bags of food.

"Evening," said Charlie.

"Hi," said Lucy and Hazel.

They unpacked the shopping and settled at the table with a cup of tea and a doughnut.

"I feel crap," said Charlie, "going to bed."

"Okay," said Hazel, "have a good sleep. You'll feel much better in the morning."

"I hope so," replied Charlie, "night."

Catherine and Charlie lay in bed. Catherine slept soundly…. pregnancy was no picnic. Charlie stared into the darkness…… body exhausted, mind alert.

"What if that dizzy spell was the start of something serious?"

His heartbeat increased. Breathing became rapid and shallow. Head pounded on the pillow, throbbing and intense. The voices in the kitchen were little more than an incoherent babble.

"Be sensible," he pleaded, "what's the point of worrying about something that'll probably never happen?"

A CRY FOR EVER

He managed a degree of control.

"Just live your life," he urged, "and don't let anything ruin it."

After twenty-five minutes, normal anxiety was resumed.

"A dizzy spell when standing too quickly is perfectly normal," he assured.

Charlie lay still, listening to Catherine's soft breathing.

"Best thing to do," he decided, "try to live your life normally, and try not to let anything ruin it."

Movement in the kitchen. He heard the key turn in the lock.

"The back door is locked," he thought," that's one less worry."

He rolled onto his front, careful not to disturb Catherine.

"Dizzy spell," he pondered, "nothing serious. No worries."

An hour later, anxiety normal, Charlie drifted into a restful sleep. Rest and recuperation….. freedom from OCD.

Tuesday, November the seventh dawned bright and clear. Birds chirped outside the window, a slight breeze rustled in the trees, a dog barked in the distance…… in fact, everything was as normal. The alarm bleeped at seven o'clock. Every minute, bleep, bleep, louder and louder. Without attention, it wasn't going to stop. Bleeps burst into Charlie's dream. He stirred, reluctantly pulled from his safe haven. He resisted, preferring dreamland to reality, and pulled the duvet over his head.

"Don't want to get up," he decided, ignoring the alarm, "what time is it?"

He snuggled under the duvet.

"What day is it?"

He closed his eyes, wishing the bloody alarm would self-destruct.

"Fucking hell," he realised, "it's today baby will be born."

He leapt out his pit. Adrenalin was far more effective than any alarm. He threw on a jumper and dungarees before clouting the bleeping clock. He must have hit the right button, as the irritating noise finally stopped.

"Catherine," he whispered, "wake up. Today's the day. We've got to get ready."

"What?"

"It's today," repeated Charlie, "you're having a Caesarean."

"Blimey," said Catherine, wide awake, "what's the time?"

"Just after seven," answered Charlie, "so we've got about an hour to get sorted."

"Okay," said Catherine, climbing from the bed, "I'll just use the bathroom."

At quarter to eight, Catherine and Charlie sat at the kitchen table, waiting for Anna.

"I really hope she gets here on time," said Charlie, "she's not famous for her punctuality."

"Don't panic," replied Catherine, "I'm sure she'll be here."

"Hope so," said Charlie, "cause Lucy and Hazel left early for work."

"Calm down," urged Catherine.

"Hope Tiger's okay," said Charlie.

"She'll be fine," replied Catherine, "she looked really happy when we dropped her at Linda's last night."

"I just worry," said Charlie.

A car pulled up outside the house.

"One less thing for you to worry about," said Catherine, "it sounds like Anna is early."

"Thank fuck for that," said Charlie, standing up, "have you got everything you need?"

"I have," replied Catherine, picking up her small bag, "let's get going."

They arrived before nine, met Catherine's mum at the entrance and headed for maternity. Shown to a room, they were greeted by the midwife.

"Will you be attending the Caesarean, Charlie?"

"Sorry?"

"If you want," she explained, "you can be in the operating room for the birth."

"Oh," muttered Charlie, "I really don't mind if Catherine's mum would like to watch, instead."

"That'd be good," added Catherine.

"I'd love to," said her mum.

Checks were completed, time passed in a haze, then Catherine was taken to the operating room with her mum in close attendance. Charlie and Anna sat and waited.

"Do you want a boy or a girl?"

"Not bothered," answered Charlie, "as long as it's healthy. Think that's what I'm supposed to say."

"Decided on names?"

"Colin," answered Charlie, "or Caroline."

"Oh," said Anna.

A CRY FOR EVER

An hour passed. Anna seemed more anxious than Charlie. Expectant fatherhood is easy when OCD has already hardened you.

"Shouldn't be much longer," said Anna.

"Hope not," replied Charlie, "but they've got to clean the baby, then stitch up Catherine......"

"Catherine didn't seem nervous," said Anna.

"No, she was fine," replied Charlie, "bloody brave. I'd have been shitting myself."

"Me too," said Anna.

"Are you and Sam going to have children?"

"I'd like to," replied Anna, "but I think Sam's firing blanks."

"Oh," said Charlie, "he told you that?"

"Well," answered Anna, "his ex-wife couldn't get pregnant after years of trying."

"Maybe she had a problem."

"Don't think so," said Anna, "she had two kids from a previous relationship."

"Oh," said Charlie, "doesn't look very promising."

"So," continued Anna, "I think Sam has convinced himself that he doesn't want children."

"I see."

The door open. Catherine's bed was wheeled into the room. A few steps behind, Catherine's mum cradled a tiny bundle. She walked over to Charlie and gently laid the newborn baby in his arms. The blanket, wrapped around the delicate frame, kept baby warm and clean.

"Wow," murmured Charlie, gazing at his creation, "what is......."

"A girl."

"Hello, Caroline," said Charlie, "glad you made it."

"Congratulations," said Anna.

Baby Caroline dozed, oblivious to the excitement caused by her presence.

"It's hard work being born," said the midwife.

"Yeah," replied Charlie, "guess so."

"Congratulations, she's perfect."

Charlie held the baby, vowing to love and protect her. The war on OCD - reinforcements had arrived. Charlie carefully placed the new baby on her mother's chest. Catherine's hands supported the infant......a life valued above her own.

"Go and have a cry," suggested the midwife, smiling at

Charlie.

"I'll settle for a fag," replied Charlie, walking to the door, "be back in a minute."

He trotted along the corridor, joyfully planning an amazing future. The sun's rays, high in the south, flooded through the windows. Light flickered across the sterile walls. Two nurses, laughing and joking, headed for maternity.

"It's strange," pondered Charlie, quickening his step, "when you're happy so is everyone else. Smile and the world smiles with you."

Two porters, little and large, carefully negotiated a safe passage for a bedridden patient. Charlie glanced at the lady as he passed. An old lady ravaged by illness. Face swollen, bruising evident, life sapping away.

"What if you were responsible for doing that? Look at the effects of a serious disease. Would any child be proud of a parent capable of something like that? Disease can ruin your ability to care for your children. Your life could be destroyed!"

Relentless ideas monopolising a situation. An opportunist seizing the moment. Charlie's heart raced and breathing quickened. He resisted an overwhelming urge to vomit on the floor. Numb legs caused an unsteady gait. Folded arms provided little reassurance. Visual disturbance added to his anxiety.

"Got to get the fuck away," he panicked, stumbling along the corridor, "there won't be so many people outside the hospital."

He passed through reception, a sea of unfamiliar faces heightening his anxiety. The automatic doors opened......... sweet relief. He crossed the road, narrowly avoiding a speeding ambulance, and flopped onto a concrete step. He checked his surroundings...... all clear.

"Calm down," he urged, "it'll be okay."

Easier said than done. Heart rate attempted a world record. Breathing like an old man with emphysema. Charlie's head dropped between his knees. Retching like a teenager on an alcohol-fuelled birthday bash. The clock was ticking...........

"Come on," he pleaded, "take control."

He'd been squatting on the step for nearly thirty minutes.

"Feel better," he decided, "they'll be wondering what's

happened."

He stood up, overwhelmed by a sense of hopelessness.

"Bloody hell," he muttered, "everything is shit. Eighteen years..... fucked-up after an hour!"

A solitary tear tricked down his cheek. A cloud covered the sun, east of the hospital. He trudged towards the entrance. Would it always be like this? For ever?

Printed in the United Kingdom
by Lightning Source UK Ltd.
124164UK00001B/175-183/A